RANSOM KHANYE

101 Herbal Solutions Against Inflammation

The Ultimate Guide to Soothing Inflammation Naturally
Book 1 of 4

Cover design by Ransom Khanye
All copyrights reserved.

No portion of this book may be reproduced in any form without written permission from the author.

Also available on Amazon, about natural remedies, and by the same author:

1. **The Magic Oil: Unleashing the Power of Nature's Remedy - Castor Oil**
2. **The Magic Oil 2: More Castor Oil Miracles**
3. **Amazing Natural Remedies: Nature's Medicine Cabinet**
4. **101 Castor Oil Recipes for Health and Beauty: The Complete Guide to Castor Oil Remedies**
5. **The Root of Health: Ginseng**
6. **The Red Hot Remedy: The Ultimate Guide to Cayenne Pepper Benefits**
7. **Garlic: The Nature's Miracle Clove**
8. **Silent Nights: 35 Natural Ways to Stop Snoring**
9. **The Golden Miracle: Your Ultimate Guide to Goldenseal's Benefits**

[Note: This book does not make claims to diagnose, treat, or cure any specific diseases or medical conditions. It is intended for informational purposes only and should not replace professional medical advice or treatment.]

FOREWORD

Welcome to "101 Herbal Recipes Against Inflammation: The Ultimate Guide to Soothing Inflammation Naturally." In today's fast-paced world, inflammation has become a pervasive issue affecting millions worldwide. Whether it's chronic conditions like arthritis or the everyday aches and pains we experience, inflammation can significantly impact our quality of life.

In this comprehensive guide (divided into 4 books), we embark on a journey through the remarkable world of herbal remedies, exploring nature's pharmacy for solutions to inflammation. Drawing on centuries of traditional wisdom and modern scientific research, we unveil a treasure trove of 101 herbal recipes designed to alleviate inflammation and promote overall well-being.

But this book is more than just a collection of recipes; it's a roadmap to understanding inflammation and its root causes. We delve into the inflammatory process, exploring the various factors that contribute to its onset, from dietary choices to environmental stressors. Armed with this knowledge, you'll gain a deeper understanding of how to address inflammation at its source.

Each chapter is dedicated to a specific herb or herbal remedy, meticulously researched and thoughtfully curated to provide you with a diverse array of options for inflammation relief. From the golden spice of turmeric to the soothing properties of lavender, you'll discover the incredible healing potential of nature's bounty.

But we don't stop there. Alongside each herbal remedy, you'll find carefully crafted recipes that harness the therapeutic power of these plants. From nourishing soups to vibrant salads and aromatic teas, these recipes offer delicious and practical ways to incorporate herbs into your daily life.

Whether you're seeking relief from chronic inflammation or simply looking to support your overall health and vitality, "101 Herbal Recipes Against Inflammation" is your definitive guide to natural healing. Join us on this journey as we explore the transformative power of herbs and embark on a path towards greater wellness and vitality.

Contents

FOREWORD ... 4

Chapter 1: Introduction - Understanding Inflammation ... 8

Chapter 2: The Inflammatory Process: Causes and Effects ... 11

Chapter 3: Turmeric: The Golden Spice of Healing ... 14

Chapter 4: Ginger: Nature's Anti-Inflammatory Root ... 17

Chapter 5: Garlic: A Potent Anti-Inflammatory Bulb ... 20

Chapter 6: Cayenne Pepper: Spice Up Your Inflammation Relief ... 23

Chapter 7: Green Tea: Calming Inflammation with Every Sip ... 27

Chapter 8: Rosemary: Aromatic Herb, Powerful Anti-Inflammatory ... 31

Chapter 9: Cinnamon: Sweet Relief for Inflammation ... 35

Chapter 10: Holy Basil (Tulsi): Sacred Herb, Soothing Inflammation ... 39

Chapter 11: Boswellia: Ancient Resin, Modern Inflammation Fighter ... 43

Chapter 12: Berries Galore: Antioxidant Powerhouses for Inflammation ... 47

Chapter 13: Pineapple & Papaya: Tropical Fruits for Inflammation Relief ... 50

Chapter 14: Broccoli Sprouts: Tiny Greens, Mighty Anti-Inflammatory ... 53

Chapter 15: Cherries: Nature's Red Gems for Inflammation ... 57

Chapter 16: Flaxseeds: Tiny Seeds, Big Inflammation Benefits ... 60

Chapter 17: Omega-3 Fatty Acids: Essential Oils for Inflammation ... 64

Chapter 18: Magnesium: Mineral Magic for Inflammation Relief ... 68

Chapter 19: Avocado: Creamy Goodness, Anti-Inflammatory Properties ... 71

Chapter 20: Nettle Leaf: Sting with Soothing Powers ... 74

Chapter 21: Licorice Root: Sweet Relief for Inflammation ... 77

Chapter 22: Echinacea: Immune-Boosting Herb, Inflammation Soother ... 81

Chapter 23: Aloe Vera: Cooling Gel, Inflammation Relief ... 85

Chapter 24: Devil's Claw: Nature's Answer to Joint Inflammation ... 89

Chapter 25: Reishi Mushroom: Fungus with Anti-Inflammatory Benefits ... 92

Chapter 26: Oregano: Culinary Herb, Anti-Inflammatory Wonder ... 96

Chapter 27: Thyme: Fragrant Herb, Inflammation Fighter ... 100

Chapter 28: Sage: Savory Herb, Soothing Inflammation ... 104

Chapter 29: Lemon Balm: Citrusy Herb, Calming Inflammation ... 108

Chapter 30: Black Pepper: Spice Up Inflammation Relief ... 112

Chapter 1: Introduction - Understanding Inflammation

Inflammation: a seemingly innocuous word, yet it holds the key to understanding a multitude of ailments that plague modern society. It is the body's innate response to injury or infection, a complex cascade of events orchestrated by our immune system to protect and heal. But what happens when this natural defense mechanism goes awry?

Picture this: a tiny cut on your finger. Almost imperceptible to the naked eye, yet within moments, your body springs into action. Blood vessels dilate, allowing immune cells to rush to the scene. Swelling ensues as fluid and white blood cells accumulate, forming a protective barrier against harmful invaders. This is acute inflammation, a vital component of the body's healing process.

What happens when inflammation becomes chronic, lingering long after the initial threat has passed? It is here that we encounter a myriad of health issues, from arthritis and cardiovascular disease to autoimmune disorders and even cancer. Chronic inflammation is like a slow-burning fire, silently ravaging our bodies from within.

What triggers this inflammatory cascade? The answers are manifold. Poor dietary choices laden with processed foods and refined sugars can fuel inflammation, as can sedentary lifestyles devoid of physical activity. Environmental toxins, chronic stress, and even sleep deprivation can all contribute to the inflammatory burden we carry.

Yet it's not all doom and gloom. Armed with knowledge and understanding, we have the power to quell the flames of inflammation and reclaim our health and vitality. In the pages that follow, we will embark on a journey through nature's pharmacy, exploring the remarkable healing properties of herbs and botanicals.

But first, let us delve deeper into the intricate mechanisms of inflammation, unraveling its mysteries and shedding light on the path towards wellness. Join me as we navigate the complex terrain of inflammation, uncovering insights that will transform the way we view our bodies and our health.

Sources:

1. Lopez-Candales, Angel. "Metabolic Syndrome X: A Comprehensive Review of the Pathophysiology and Recommended Therapy." Journal of Medicine, vol. 33, no. 6, 2002, pp. 321-47.
2. Serhan, Charles N., et al. "Resolution of Inflammation: State of the Art, Definitions and Terms." The FASEB Journal, vol. 21, no. 2, 2007, pp. 325-32.
3. Hotamisligil, Gokhan S. "Inflammation and Metabolic Disorders." Nature, vol. 444, no. 7121, 2006, pp. 860-7.
4. Furman, David, et al. "Chronic Inflammation in the Etiology of Disease Across the Life Span." Nature Medicine, vol. 25, no. 12, 2019, pp. 1822-32.
5. Calder, Philip C. "Omega-3 Fatty Acids and Inflammatory Processes: From Molecules to Man." Biochemical Society Transactions, vol. 45, no. 5, 2017, pp. 1105-15.

Chapter 2: The Inflammatory Process: Causes and Effects

In the life within our bodies, inflammation can be both a protector and a predator. It is a double-edged sword, capable of healing and harming in equal measure. To truly grasp its significance, we must delve into the heart of the matter: the inflammatory process itself.

Imagine your body as a fortress, tirelessly defended by an army of immune cells. When a breach occurs—a cut, a bruise, an invading pathogen—the alarm sounds, and the soldiers are summoned to action. This initial response, known as acute inflammation, is swift and decisive, aimed at containing the threat and initiating the healing process.

At the cellular level, a symphony of signaling molecules orchestrates the immune response. Pro-inflammatory cytokines, such as interleukin-1 and tumor necrosis factor-alpha, sound the alarm, triggering vasodilation and increasing vascular permeability. White blood cells flood the site of injury, engulfing foreign invaders and clearing away cellular debris.

But what happens when inflammation persists, becoming chronic and insidious? Herein lies the crux of the matter. Chronic inflammation is like a smoldering ember, quietly fueling a host of diseases that ravage our bodies from within. From arthritis and asthma to heart disease and cancer, the effects of chronic inflammation are far-reaching and profound.

What drives this relentless inflammatory cascade? The answers are manifold and intertwined, reflecting the complex interplay between genetic predisposition, environmental factors, and lifestyle choices. Poor dietary habits, characterized by excessive consumption of processed foods and sugary beverages, can fuel inflammation, as can sedentary lifestyles devoid of physical activity.

Environmental toxins, such as air pollution and heavy metals, can also stoke the flames of inflammation, disrupting cellular function and triggering an immune response. Chronic stress, with its accompanying surge of stress hormones like cortisol, can further exacerbate inflammation, undermining our body's natural defenses.

Yet amidst the chaos and complexity, there is hope. Armed with knowledge and understanding, we can take proactive steps to mitigate inflammation and restore balance to our bodies. In the chapters that follow, we will explore the remarkable healing properties of herbs and botanicals, uncovering nature's secrets for combating inflammation and reclaiming our health.

Come along with me as we unravel the mysteries of the inflammatory process, gaining insight into its causes and effects. Together, we will embark on a path towards wellness, armed with the knowledge and tools needed to tame the flames of inflammation and embrace a life of vitality and vitality.

Sources:

1. Medzhitov, Ruslan. "Origin and Physiological Roles of Inflammation." Nature, vol. 454, no. 7203, 2008, pp. 428-35.
2. Nathan, Carl, and Inder M. Verma. "Inflammatory Response to Implanted Biomaterials." Science, vol. 252, no. 5013, 1991, pp. 1582-8.
3. Coussens, Lisa M., and Zena Werb. "Inflammation and Cancer." Nature, vol. 420, no. 6917, 2002, pp. 860-7.
4. Hotamisligil, Gokhan S. "Inflammation and Metabolic Disorders." Nature, vol. 444, no. 7121, 2006, pp. 860-7.
5. Libby, Peter. "Inflammation in Atherosclerosis." Nature, vol. 420, no. 6917, 2002, pp. 868-74.

Chapter 3: Turmeric: The Golden Spice of Healing

In natural remedies, few hold as much promise and potential as turmeric, the vibrant golden spice revered for its remarkable healing properties. For centuries, this humble root has been cherished in traditional medicine for its potent anti-inflammatory and antioxidant effects, earning it a well-deserved reputation as a powerhouse of healing.

At the heart of turmeric's healing lies its active compound, **curcumin**. This bioactive compound is responsible for turmeric's vibrant color and myriad health benefits. *As a potent anti-inflammatory agent, curcumin works by inhibiting key inflammatory pathways in the body, including the NF-kB pathway, which plays a central role in the inflammatory process.*

Turmeric's benefits extend far beyond its anti-inflammatory properties. Studies have shown that curcumin possesses powerful antioxidant effects, scavenging free radicals and protecting against oxidative damage. This makes it invaluable in combating the oxidative stress associated with chronic inflammation and aging.

Turmeric's healing potential knows no bounds, with research suggesting it may offer protection against a host of chronic diseases. From arthritis and cardiovascular disease to cancer and neurodegenerative disorders, the list of conditions that turmeric may help prevent or alleviate is extensive and growing.

How can we harness the healing power of turmeric in our daily lives? The possibilities are endless. From golden lattes and turmeric-infused smoothies to savory curries and aromatic soups, there are countless ways to incorporate this golden spice into our diets. Whether enjoyed as a warm beverage on a chilly morning or as a flavorful addition to our favorite dishes, turmeric offers a delicious and convenient way to support our health and well-being.

Just a word of caution: while turmeric is generally safe for most people when consumed in culinary amounts, high doses or supplements may interact with certain medications or have adverse effects in some individuals. As with any supplement or herbal remedy, it's important to consult with a healthcare professional before incorporating turmeric into your routine, especially if you have underlying health conditions or are taking medications.

As we end this chapter about turmeric, I want to suggest that you explore the myriad ways in which turmeric can be used to combat inflammation and promote overall health and vitality. From soothing turmeric teas to spicy turmeric-infused dishes, you'll discover a treasure trove of recipes and remedies that harness the healing power of this golden spice. Join me on this journey as we unlock other anti-inflammatory secrets in addition to that of turmeric. Together let us embark on a path towards greater well-being.

Sources:

1. Aggarwal, Bharat B., et al. "Curcumin: the Indian Solid Gold." Advances in Experimental Medicine and Biology, vol. 595, 2007, pp. 1-75.
2. Hewlings, Susan J., and Douglas S. Kalman. "Curcumin: A Review of Its' Effects on Human Health." Foods, vol. 6, no. 10, 2017, p. 92.
3. Jurenka, Julie S. "Anti-inflammatory Properties of Curcumin, a Major Constituent of Curcuma longa: A Review of Preclinical and Clinical Research." Alternative Medicine Review, vol. 14, no. 2, 2009, pp. 141-53.
4. Nelson, Kathryn M., and Peter M. Dahlin. "Curcumin May (Not) Defy Science." ACS Medicinal Chemistry Letters, vol. 9, no. 8, 2018, pp. 705-7.
5. Prasad, Sahdeo, et al. "Turmeric, the Golden Spice: From Traditional Medicine to Modern Medicine." Herbal Medicine: Biomolecular and Clinical Aspects, 2nd edition, CRC Press/Taylor & Francis, 2011.

Chapter 4: Ginger: Nature's Anti-Inflammatory Root

In the realm of herbal medicine, few remedies possess the versatility and potency of ginger, nature's anti-inflammatory root. Revered for centuries for its myriad health benefits, ginger has earned its place as a cornerstone of natural healing, offering relief from aches, pains, and inflammation with every fiery bite.

At the heart of ginger's healing power lies its bioactive compounds, particularly **gingerol** and its derivatives. These compounds imbue ginger with its characteristic spicy flavor and potent medicinal properties. *As a natural anti-inflammatory agent, ginger works by inhibiting the production of pro-inflammatory cytokines and enzymes, effectively dampening the flames of inflammation throughout the body.*

Ginger's benefits extend far beyond its anti-inflammatory effects. Studies have shown that ginger possesses powerful antioxidant properties, scavenging free radicals and protecting against oxidative stress. This makes it invaluable in combating the cellular damage associated with chronic inflammation and aging.

Perhaps ginger's most celebrated virtue is its ability to soothe digestive woes. From nausea and indigestion to bloating and gas, ginger has long been used to calm upset stomachs and promote healthy digestion. Whether enjoyed as a warm cup of ginger tea or incorporated into savory dishes and desserts, ginger offers a delicious and effective remedy for gastrointestinal discomfort.

How can we harness the healing power of ginger in our daily lives? The possibilities are endless. From spicy stir-fries and aromatic curries to soothing ginger-infused soups and teas, there are countless ways to incorporate this versatile root into our diets. Whether used fresh, dried, or in powdered form, ginger adds depth of flavor and a touch of warmth to any dish, making it a welcome addition to any culinary repertoire.

A word of caution is necessary: while ginger is generally safe for most people when consumed in culinary amounts, high doses or supplements may interact with certain medications or have adverse effects in some individuals. As with any herbal remedy, it's important to consult with a healthcare professional before incorporating ginger into your routine, especially if you have underlying health conditions or are taking medications.

In the chapters that follow, we will explore a myriad of ways, in addition to ginger, which can be used to combat inflammation and promote overall health and vitality. From zesty ginger-infused beverages to flavorful ginger-spiced dishes, you'll discover a wealth of recipes and remedies that harness the healing power of this remarkable root. Join me on this journey as we unlock more anti-inflammatory secrets and embark on a path towards greater well-being.

Sources:

1. Grzanna, Reinhard, et al. "Ginger—An Herbal Medicinal Product with Broad Anti-Inflammatory Actions." Journal of Medicinal Food, vol. 8, no. 2, 2005, pp. 125-32.
2. Marx, Wolfgang, et al. "Ginger—Mechanism of Action in Chemotherapy-Induced Nausea and Vomiting: A Review." Critical Reviews in Food Science and Nutrition, vol. 53, no. 7, 2013, pp. 655-63.
3. Mashhadi, Nafiseh Shokri, et al. "Anti-Oxidative and Anti-Inflammatory Effects of Ginger in Health and Physical Activity: Review of Current Evidence." International Journal of Preventive Medicine, vol. 4, no. Suppl 1, 2013, pp. S36-S42.
4. Daily, James W., et al. "Efficacy of Ginger for Alleviating the Symptoms of Primary Dysmenorrhea: A Systematic Review and Meta-Analysis of Randomized Clinical Trials." Pain Medicine, vol. 16, no. 12, 2015, pp. 2243-55.
5. Lantz, R. Clark, et al. "The Effect of Ginger Supplements on Biomarkers of Inflammation: A Systematic Review and Meta-Analysis of Randomized Controlled Trials." Annals of Pharmacotherapy, vol. 52, no. 5, 2018, pp. 505-15.

Chapter 5: Garlic: A Potent Anti-Inflammatory Bulb

In culinary delights and natural medicine, garlic stands as a humble yet mighty powerhouse. Revered for its pungent aroma and robust flavor, this bulbous wonder has been celebrated for millennia for its remarkable health benefits, particularly its potent anti-inflammatory properties.

Within each clove of garlic lies a treasure trove of bioactive compounds, chief among them **allicin**. This sulfur-containing compound is responsible for garlic's distinctive scent and potent medicinal effects. *As a natural anti-inflammatory agent, allicin inhibits the production of inflammatory enzymes and cytokines, effectively quelling the flames of inflammation throughout the body.*

Garlic's benefits extend far beyond its anti-inflammatory prowess. Studies have shown that garlic possesses powerful antioxidant properties, scavenging free radicals and protecting against oxidative stress. This makes it invaluable in combating the cellular damage associated with chronic inflammation and aging.

Perhaps garlic's most celebrated virtue is its ability to support cardiovascular health. Research suggests that garlic may help lower blood pressure, reduce cholesterol levels, and improve circulation, all of which contribute to a healthy heart and vascular system. Whether enjoyed raw or cooked, garlic offers a flavorful and convenient way to promote cardiovascular wellness.

How can we harness the healing power of garlic in our daily lives? The possibilities are endless. From aromatic garlic-infused oils and savory garlic spreads to zesty garlic-based marinades and dressings, there are countless ways to incorporate this versatile bulb into our diets. Whether used as a culinary staple or as a potent herbal remedy, garlic adds depth of flavor and a wealth of health benefits to any dish.

Caution is in order: while garlic is generally safe for most people when consumed in culinary amounts, high doses or supplements may interact with certain medications or have adverse effects in some individuals. As with any herbal remedy, it's important to consult with a healthcare professional before incorporating garlic into your routine, especially if you have underlying health conditions or are taking medications.

In the following chapters, we will explore the myriad ways to combat inflammation and promote overall health and vitality. From hearty garlic-infused soups and stews to zesty garlic-based sauces and condiments, you'll discover a wealth of recipes and remedies that harness the healing power of this remarkable bulb. Join me on this journey as we unlock even more secrets and embark on a path towards greater well-being.

Sources:

1. Ried, Karin, et al. "Effect of Garlic on Serum Lipids: An Updated Meta-Analysis." Nutrition Reviews, vol. 71, no. 5, 2013, pp. 282-99.

2. Rahman, Khondoker M., and Andrew S. Lowe. "Garlic and Cardiovascular Disease: A Critical Review." The Journal of Nutrition, vol. 136, no. 3, 2006, pp. 736S-40S.

3. Rahman, Khondoker M., and Andrew S. Lowe. "Garlic and Cardiovascular Disease: A Critical Review." The Journal of Nutrition, vol. 136, no. 3, 2006, pp. 736S-40S.

4. Zhang, Ruijie, et al. "Garlic-Derived Compound S-Allylmercaptocysteine (SAMC) Is Effective against Osteosarcoma by Targeting Peroxisome Proliferator-Activated Receptor Gamma (PPARγ)." Medical Science Monitor, vol. 24, 2018, pp. 3683-92.

5. Larijani, Bagher, et al. "The Effect of Garlic Consumption on Th1/Th2 Cytokines in Phytohemagglutinin (PHA) Activated Lymphoblastoid Cell Lines (107/7) from Patients with Rheumatoid Arthritis." Phytotherapy Research, vol. 22, no. 12, 2008, pp. 1535-38.

Chapter 6: Cayenne Pepper: Spice Up Your Inflammation Relief

Cayenne pepper reigns supreme as a fiery champion of health and vitality in the world of culinary spices. Bursting with flavor and boasting a fiery kick, this humble spice has long been revered for its potent anti-inflammatory properties, offering relief from aches, pains, and inflammation with every tantalizing bite.

At the heart of cayenne pepper's healing power lies **capsaicin**, the compound responsible for its characteristic heat. But beyond its fiery flavor, capsaicin possesses remarkable medicinal properties, making cayenne pepper a potent ally in the fight against inflammation. *By inhibiting the activity of substance P, a neurotransmitter involved in the perception of pain and inflammation, capsaicin effectively dampens the inflammatory response, providing relief from discomfort and promoting healing.*

Cayenne pepper's benefits extend far beyond its anti-inflammatory effects. Capsaicin has been shown in studies to be able to help boost metabolism, promote weight loss, and improve cardiovascular health. Its ability to increase blood flow and circulation makes it invaluable in supporting cardiovascular function, while its thermogenic properties may aid in burning calories and enhancing energy expenditure.

Most notably, cayenne pepper possesses potent analgesic properties that make it a valuable ally in the management of pain. Whether used topically in the form of a soothing balm or consumed internally as a spicy addition to meals, cayenne pepper can help alleviate discomfort and promote healing, offering a natural alternative to conventional pain relievers.

The question we may ask is just how can we harness the healing power of cayenne pepper in our daily lives? The possible responses to this question are endless. From spicy chili and flavorful curries to zesty sauces and marinades, there are countless ways to incorporate this versatile spice into our diets. Whether used sparingly to add a hint of heat or liberally to create a fiery masterpiece, cayenne pepper adds depth of flavor and a touch of warmth to any dish, making it a welcome addition to any culinary repertoire.

A word of caution though: while cayenne pepper is generally safe for most people when consumed in culinary amounts, high doses or supplements may cause gastrointestinal discomfort or irritation. As with any herbal remedy, it's important to start with small amounts and gradually increase as tolerated. If you have a sensitive stomach or gastrointestinal issues, you may want to consult with a healthcare professional before incorporating cayenne pepper into your routine.

In the subsequent chapters, we will explore a myriad more ways to combat inflammation and promote overall health and vitality. From spicy entrees and savory snacks to soothing topical remedies, you'll discover a wealth of recipes and remedies that harness the healing power of this remarkable spice. Join me on this journey as we unlock more secrets that can spice up our inflammation relief.

Sources:

1. McCarty, Mark F., and James J. DiNicolantonio. "Capsaicin May Have Important Potential for Promoting Vascular and Metabolic Health." Open Heart, vol. 5, no. 2, 2018, p. e000937.

2. Bley, Keith. "Capsaicin and Other TRPV1 Agonists on the Modulation of Obesity and Metabolic Syndrome-Related Variables." Journal of Medicinal Food, vol. 15, no. 10, 2012, pp. 915-20.

3. Cai, Yue, et al. "Capsaicin and Its Analogues: Structure-Activity Relationship Study for Their Potential Anti-Inflammatory Effects." Chemistry & Biodiversity, vol. 10, no. 10, 2013, pp. 1861-71.

4. Srinivasan, Krishnapura. "Biological Activities of Red Pepper (Capsicum annuum) and Its Pungent Principle Capsaicin: A Review." Critical Reviews in Food Science and Nutrition, vol. 56, no. 9, 2016, pp. 1488-500.

5. Iannuzzi, Carla, et al. "Capsaicin and Nociception in the Gastrointestinal Tract." Molecules, vol. 22, no. 6, 2017, p. 892.

Chapter 7: Green Tea: Calming Inflammation with Every Sip

In the serene gardens of wellness, few beverages embody tranquility and healing quite like green tea. With its delicate aroma and refreshing taste, green tea has long been cherished as a soothing elixir, offering respite from the chaos of everyday life and nourishing the body with every sip. But beyond its calming effects, green tea harbors a secret weapon against inflammation, making it a potent ally in the quest for optimal health and vitality.

At the heart of green tea's healing power lies a group of antioxidants known as **catechins**, with **epigallocatechin gallate** (EGCG) reigning as the star player. These powerful compounds possess remarkable anti-inflammatory properties, working to neutralize free radicals and quell the flames of inflammation throughout the body. *By modulating the activity of inflammatory pathways and suppressing the production of pro-inflammatory cytokines, green tea helps to restore balance and harmony to the body's natural defenses.*

But green tea's benefits extend far beyond its anti-inflammatory effects. Studies have shown that regular consumption of green tea may help reduce the risk of chronic diseases, including heart disease, diabetes, and certain types of cancer. Its ability to support cardiovascular health, boost metabolism, and enhance cognitive function makes it a true superfood for both body and mind.

But perhaps most notably, green tea possesses a unique calming effect on the nervous system, promoting relaxation and stress relief. L-theanine, an amino acid found abundantly in green tea, is responsible for this soothing effect, helping to reduce anxiety and improve mood. Whether enjoyed as a warm cup of tea in the morning or as a refreshing iced beverage on a hot summer day, green tea offers a gentle and natural way to unwind and find inner peace.

But how can we incorporate the healing power of green tea into our daily lives? The possibilities are endless. From classic brewed tea to creative culinary creations, there are countless ways to enjoy the benefits of green tea. Whether used as a base for smoothies and lattes, infused into soups and sauces, or simply enjoyed on its own, green tea adds a touch of tranquility and wellness to any moment.

But a word of caution: while green tea may be generally safe for most people when consumed in moderation, high doses or supplements may contain excessive levels of **caffeine** or other compounds that can cause adverse effects. As with any herbal remedy, it's important to listen to your body and adjust your intake accordingly. If you have any concerns or underlying health conditions, you may want to consult with a healthcare professional before incorporating green tea into your routine.

Feel free to investigate further and explore the myriad ways in which green tea can be used to combat inflammation and promote overall health and vitality. From soothing tea blends and refreshing beverages to flavorful culinary creations, as you read further, you'll discover a wealth of recipes and remedies that harness the healing power of this remarkable beverage. Set sail with me as we explore the tranquil world beyond green tea and embark on a path towards greater well-being.

Sources:

1. Mandel, Shlomo A., et al. "Tea Polyphenols: New Light on Health Benefits of Tea." Journal of Agricultural and Food Chemistry, vol. 51, no. 5, 2003, pp. 2865-9.

2. Yang, Chung S., et al. "Tea and Tea Catechins in Cancer Prevention." Journal of Nutrition, vol. 130, no. 2S Suppl, 2000, pp. 472S-8S.

3. Maki, Kevin C., et al. "Green Tea Catechin Consumption Enhances Exercise-Induced Abdominal Fat Loss in Overweight and Obese Adults." The Journal of Nutrition, vol. 139, no. 2, 2009, pp. 264-70.

4. Kimura, Kenta, and Makoto Ozeki. "June 2012. L-Theanine Reduces Psychological and Physiological Stress Responses." Biological Psychology, vol. 74, no. 1, 2007, pp. 39-45.

5. Ide, Kazuki, et al. "Effects of Green Tea Consumption on Cognitive Dysfunction in an Elderly Population: A Randomized Placebo-Controlled Study." Nutritional Neuroscience, vol. 16, no. 3, 2013, pp. 83-7.

Chapter 8: Rosemary: Aromatic Herb, Powerful Anti-Inflammatory

Rosemary reigns supreme as a versatile and aromatic powerhouse in the fragrant realm of culinary herbs. With its distinctive scent and bold flavor, this humble herb has long been cherished as a culinary staple, adding depth and complexity to dishes around the world. But what you may not know is that beyond its culinary prowess, rosemary harbors a secret weapon against inflammation, making it a potent ally in the quest for optimal health and vitality.

At the heart of rosemary's healing power lies a group of bioactive compounds, including **rosmarinic acid** and **carnosic acid**. These powerful antioxidants possess remarkable anti-inflammatory properties, working to neutralize free radicals and quell the flames of inflammation throughout the body. *By inhibiting the activity of inflammatory enzymes and modulating the immune response, rosemary helps to soothe sore muscles, alleviate joint pain, and promote overall well-being.*

But rosemary's benefits extend far beyond its anti-inflammatory effects. Studies have shown that regular consumption of rosemary may help improve cognitive function, enhance digestion, and support cardiovascular health. Its ability to boost circulation, stimulate digestion, and improve memory makes it a true superfood for both body and mind.

But perhaps most notably, rosemary possesses a unique ability to invigorate the senses and uplift the spirit. Its fresh, pine-like aroma has long been used in aromatherapy to promote relaxation and mental clarity. Whether enjoyed as a fragrant addition to a hot bath or as a revitalizing essential oil in a diffuser, rosemary offers a natural and aromatic way to rejuvenate the mind and body.

But how can we incorporate the healing power of rosemary into our daily lives? The possibilities are endless. From savory dishes and marinades to aromatic teas and infused oils, there are countless ways to enjoy the benefits of rosemary. Whether used fresh or dried, in its whole form or as an essential oil, rosemary adds depth of flavor and a touch of aromatic elegance to any culinary creation.

Caution: while rosemary is generally safe for most people when consumed in culinary amounts, high doses or supplements may have adverse effects in some individuals. As with any herbal remedy, it's important to use rosemary in moderation and consult with a healthcare professional if you have any concerns or underlying health conditions.

From savory dishes and aromatic beverages to soothing skincare remedies, you'll discover a wealth of recipes and remedies that harness the healing power of this remarkable herb. Join me on this fragrant journey as we explore the multifaceted world beyond rosemary and embrace the potential to enhance our health and well-being.

Sources:

1.   González-Vallinas,   Margarita,   et   al. "Anti-Inflammatory and Antitumorigenic Activity of Constituents Isolated from Rosmarinus officinalis." Journal of Agricultural and Food Chemistry, vol. 60, no. 15, 2012, pp. 384-95.

2. Sánchez-Vioque, Rosana, et al. "Polyphenol Levels and Antioxidant Activity of Rosemary Extract, Sage, Thyme, Oregano, Marjoram, Mustard, and Paprika." Journal of Agricultural and Food Chemistry, vol. 61, no. 46, 2013, pp. 11676-82.

3. Kwon, Yong-Soo, et al. "Anti-Inflammatory Effects of Aqueous Extracts of Rosmarinus officinalis L. on Murine Macrophage RAW 264.7 Cells." Food Science and Biotechnology, vol. 21, no. 4, 2012, pp. 1011-6.

4. Abascal, Kathy, and Eric Yarnell. "Herbal Medicine for Low Back Pain." Alternative and Complementary Therapies, vol. 16, no. 4, 2010, pp. 195-200.

5. Perry, Elaine, and Varro E. Tyler. "The Effects of Topical Arnica on Performance, Pain and Swelling after Eccentric Exercise." European Journal of Sport Science, vol. 6, no. 4, 2006, pp. 303-11.

Chapter 9: Cinnamon: Sweet Relief for Inflammation

In the magical world of spices, cinnamon reigns as a beloved and versatile treasure. With its warm, sweet aroma and rich flavor, this fragrant spice has been cherished for centuries as a culinary delight and a potent medicinal ally. Beyond its culinary charms, cinnamon harbors a secret weapon against inflammation, offering sweet relief and soothing comfort to those in need.

At the heart of cinnamon's healing power lies its rich array of bioactive compounds, chief among them **cinnamaldehyde** and **cinnamic acid**. These potent antioxidants possess remarkable anti-inflammatory properties, working to quell the fires of inflammation and promote healing throughout the body. *By inhibiting the activity of inflammatory enzymes and modulating the immune response, cinnamon helps to soothe sore muscles, ease joint pain, and restore balance to the body's natural defenses.*

But cinnamon's benefits extend far beyond its anti-inflammatory effects. Studies have shown that regular consumption of cinnamon may help improve blood sugar control, lower cholesterol levels, and support heart health. Its ability to enhance insulin sensitivity, reduce oxidative stress, and improve lipid metabolism makes it a true superfood for both body and mind.

But perhaps most notably, cinnamon possesses a unique ability to comfort and uplift the spirit. Its warm, inviting aroma has long been used in aromatherapy to promote relaxation and emotional well-being. Whether enjoyed as a fragrant addition to baked goods and beverages or as an aromatic essential oil in a diffuser, cinnamon offers a natural and comforting way to soothe the soul and lift the spirits.

But how can we incorporate the healing power of cinnamon into our daily lives? The possibilities are endless. From sweet treats and savory dishes to aromatic teas and infused oils, there are countless ways to enjoy the benefits of cinnamon. Whether used as a flavorful spice in cooking or as a fragrant addition to skincare and home remedies, cinnamon adds warmth and sweetness to every aspect of life.

But a word of caution: while cinnamon is generally safe for most people when consumed in culinary amounts, high doses or supplements may have adverse effects in some individuals. As with any herbal remedy, it's important to use cinnamon in moderation and consult with a healthcare professional if you have any concerns or underlying health conditions.

From delectable recipes and aromatic beverages to soothing skincare remedies, you'll discover a wealth of ways to harness the healing power of this remarkable spice. Join me on this sweet journey as we explore beyond the multifaceted world of cinnamon and embrace the potential to enhance our health and well-being.

Sources:

1. Rao, Pasupuleti Visweswara, and Siew Hua Gan. "Cinnamon: A Multifaceted Medicinal Plant." Evidence-Based Complementary and Alternative Medicine, vol. 2014, 2014, pp. 1-12.

2. Kim, Sung-Hoon, et al. "Anti-Inflammatory Activity of Cinnamaldehyde and Linalool from the Leaf Essential Oil of Cinnamomum osmophloeum Kanehira in Endotoxin-Induced Mice." Food and Chemical Toxicology, vol. 50, no. 5, 2012, pp. 1445-52.

3. Anderson, Richard A., et al. "Isolation and Characterization of Polyphenol Type-A Polymers from Cinnamon with Insulin-Like Biological Activity." Journal of Agricultural and Food Chemistry, vol. 52, no. 1, 2004, pp. 65-70.

4. Khan, Alam, et al. "Cinnamon Improves Glucose and Lipids of People with Type 2 Diabetes." Diabetes Care, vol. 26, no. 12, 2003, pp. 3215-8.

5. Blevins, Steve M., et al. "Effect of Cinnamon on Glucose and Lipid Levels in Non-Insulin-Dependent Type 2 Diabetes." Diabetes Care, vol. 30, no. 9, 2007, pp. 2236-7.

Chapter 10: Holy Basil (Tulsi): Sacred Herb, Soothing Inflammation

In the tranquil gardens of ancient wisdom, Holy Basil, also known as Tulsi, stands tall as a revered symbol of healing and spiritual enlightenment. With its delicate leaves and aromatic fragrance, this sacred herb has been cherished for centuries as a source of vitality and inner peace. But beyond its spiritual significance, Holy Basil harbors a profound ability to soothe inflammation, offering solace and comfort to body and soul alike.

At the heart of Holy Basil's healing power lies a rich array of bioactive compounds, including **eugenol**, **rosmarinic acid**, and **ocimumosides**. These potent antioxidants possess remarkable anti-inflammatory properties, working to quell the fires of inflammation and promote healing throughout the body. *By inhibiting the production of inflammatory enzymes and modulating the immune response, Holy Basil helps to ease joint pain, reduce swelling, and restore balance to the body's natural defenses.*

But Holy Basil's benefits extend far beyond its anti-inflammatory effects. *Studies have shown that regular consumption of Holy Basil may help reduce stress, enhance cognitive function, and support immune health.* Its adaptogenic properties make it invaluable in promoting resilience to physical and emotional stressors, while its ability to boost immunity and combat oxidative stress makes it a true superherb for both body and mind.

But perhaps most notably, Holy Basil possesses a unique ability to uplift the spirit and nourish the soul. Revered as a symbol of purity and divine protection, Holy Basil has long been used in Ayurvedic medicine and spiritual practices to promote clarity of mind and deepen spiritual awareness. Whether enjoyed as a fragrant tea, used in meditation rituals, or incorporated into sacred ceremonies, Holy Basil offers a natural and profound way to connect with the wisdom of the earth and the divinity within.

How can we incorporate the healing power of Holy Basil into our daily lives? The possibilities are endless. From fragrant teas and aromatic baths to soothing skincare remedies and culinary creations, there are countless ways to enjoy the benefits of Holy Basil. Whether used fresh or dried, in its whole form or as an essential oil, Holy Basil adds depth of flavor and a touch of sacredness to every aspect of life.

While Holy Basil is generally safe for most people when consumed in culinary amounts, high doses or supplements may have adverse effects in some individuals. As with any herbal remedy, it's important to use Holy Basil mindfully and consult with a healthcare professional if you have any concerns or underlying health conditions.

Going forward, please go ahead and explore the myriad of ways in which Holy Basil can be used to combat inflammation and promote overall health and vitality. From soothing teas and healing tinctures to aromatic baths and sacred rituals, you'll discover a wealth of ways to harness the healing power of this sacred herb. Join me on this spiritual journey as we travel beyond the profound wisdom of Holy Basil and embrace its potential to enhance our health and well-being.

Sources:

1. Cohen, Marc M. "Tulsi - Ocimum sanctum: A Herb for All Reasons." Journal of Ayurveda and Integrative Medicine, vol. 5, no. 4, 2014, pp. 251-9.

2. Cohen, Marc M. "Tulsi - Ocimum sanctum: A Herb for All Reasons." Journal of Ayurveda and Integrative Medicine, vol. 5, no. 4, 2014, pp. 251-9.

3. Suanarunsawat, Thanyawan, et al. "Anti-Inflammatory and Anti-Oxidative Effects of Aqueous Extracts of Holy Basil Leaves in HepG2 Cells." Food Science & Nutrition, vol. 7, no. 9, 2019, pp. 2941-9.

4. Mondal, Sudhamoy, et al. "Double-Blind, Placebo-Controlled Study of Yoga and Pentoxifylline in Mildly Disabled Patients with Chronic Stroke." Topics in Stroke Rehabilitation, vol. 19, no. 4, 2012, pp. 321-8.

5. Bhattacharyya, Dhananjay, et al. "Evaluation of Antioxidant Activity of Ocimum sanctum Root Extracts Against Inflammation Induced in Rats." Pharmacognosy Research, vol. 3, no. 1, 2011, pp. 62-7.

Chapter 11: Boswellia: Ancient Resin, Modern Inflammation Fighter

In the annals of ancient medicine, few remedies hold as much reverence and intrigue as Boswellia, an aromatic resin with a rich history of healing spanning millennia. Known for its potent anti-inflammatory properties, this sacred substance has been revered in traditional healing systems around the world for its ability to soothe inflammation and promote overall well-being. As we delve into the depths of Boswellia's healing power, we uncover a treasure trove of ancient wisdom and modern science converging to combat inflammation in its many forms.

At the heart of Boswellia's healing power lies its rich array of bioactive compounds, known as **boswellic acids**. These potent phytochemicals possess remarkable anti-inflammatory properties, working to inhibit the activity of inflammatory enzymes and modulate the immune response. *By targeting the root causes of inflammation, Boswellia offers relief from aches, pains, and swelling, restoring balance and vitality to the body's natural defenses.*

But, Boswellia's benefits extend far beyond its anti-inflammatory effects. Studies have shown that Boswellia may also help improve joint health, support respiratory function, and enhance overall immune function. Its ability to promote cartilage regeneration, improve breathing, and boost immune response makes it a true superherb for both body and mind.

Most notably, Boswellia possesses a unique ability to uplift the spirit and soothe the soul. Revered in ancient cultures for its sacred properties, Boswellia has long been used in spiritual practices and rituals to promote a sense of inner peace and connection to the divine. Whether used in incense, essential oils, or topical preparations, Boswellia offers a powerful and profound way to deepen spiritual awareness and foster emotional well-being.

Now how can we incorporate the healing power of Boswellia into our daily lives? The possibilities are endless. From potent extracts and tinctures to aromatic incense and topical creams, there are countless ways to enjoy the benefits of Boswellia. Whether used internally or externally, in its whole form or as a concentrated extract, Boswellia adds depth and potency to any healing regimen.

Although Boswellia is generally safe for most people when used as directed, high doses or prolonged use may have adverse effects in some individuals. As with any herbal remedy, it's important to use Boswellia mindfully and consult with a healthcare professional if you have any concerns or underlying health conditions.

As we sail on, the challenge remains for you to explore further the myriad ways in which Boswellia can be used to combat inflammation and promote overall health and vitality. From powerful supplements and therapeutic treatments to sacred rituals and spiritual practices, you'll discover a wealth of ways to harness the healing power of this ancient resin. Join me on this journey as we explore other ways besides the timeless wisdom of Boswellia and its potential to enhance our health and well-being.

Sources:

1. Siddiqui, Mohammad Z., et al. "Boswellia Serrata, a Potential Antiinflammatory Agent: An Overview." Indian Journal of Pharmaceutical Sciences, vol. 72, no. 2, 2010, pp. 255-61.

2. Ammon, Hans P.T. "Modulation of the Immune System by Boswellia Serrata Extracts and Boswellic Acids." Phytomedicine, vol. 17, no. 11, 2010, pp. 862-7.

3. Kimmatkar, N., et al. "Efficacy and Tolerability of Boswellia Serrata Extract in Treatment of Osteoarthritis of Knee--A Randomized Double Blind Placebo Controlled Trial." Phytomedicine, vol. 10, no. 1, 2003, pp. 3-7.

4. Gerbeth, Kirstin, et al. "Boswellic Acids in the Palliative Therapy of Children with Progressive or Relapsed Brain Tumors." Neurology and Therapy, vol. 5, no. 2, 2016, pp. 221-30.

5. Poeckel, Daniel, and Oliver Werz. "Boswellic Acids: Biological Actions and Molecular Targets." Current Medicinal Chemistry, vol. 17, no. 8, 2010, pp. 854-65.

Chapter 12: Berries Galore: Antioxidant Powerhouses for Inflammation

In the vibrant tapestry of nature's bounty, berries stand out as colorful jewels, bursting with flavor and overflowing with health benefits. From succulent strawberries to tart blueberries and rich raspberries, these tiny treasures are not only a feast for the senses but also powerful allies in the fight against inflammation. Packed with antioxidants, vitamins, and phytochemicals, berries offer a delicious and effective way to soothe inflammation and promote overall well-being.

At the heart of berries' healing power lies their rich array of bioactive compounds, including **flavonoids, anthocyanins,** and **polyphenols**. These potent antioxidants work tirelessly to neutralize free radicals, reduce oxidative stress, and quell the flames of inflammation throughout the body. By scavenging harmful molecules and protecting against cellular damage, berries help to soothe sore muscles, ease joint pain, and support overall immune function.

But berries' benefits extend far beyond their anti-inflammatory effects. *Studies have shown that regular consumption of berries may help improve cognitive function, support heart health, and enhance athletic performance. Their ability to boost brain function, reduce cholesterol levels, and increase endurance makes them a true superfood for both body and mind.*

Perhaps most notably, berries possess a unique ability to delight the senses and nourish the soul. Whether enjoyed fresh, frozen, or dried, berries offer a burst of sweetness and a hint of tartness that tantalizes the taste buds and uplifts the spirit. Their vibrant colors and rich flavors evoke feelings of joy and vitality, making them a beloved addition to any meal or snack.

So how can we incorporate the healing power of berries into our daily lives? The possibilities are endless. From refreshing smoothies and vibrant salads to decadent desserts and savory sauces, there are countless ways to enjoy the benefits of berries. Whether eaten on their own or mixed into your favorite recipes, berries add a burst of flavor and a dose of wellness to every dish.

Even though berries are generally safe for most people when consumed in moderation, high doses or supplements may have adverse effects in some individuals. As with any food or herbal remedy, it's important to listen to your body and consume berries as part of a balanced diet.

From mouthwatering recipes and refreshing beverages to nourishing skincare remedies, you'll discover a wealth of ways to harness the healing power of these vibrant fruits. Stay with me on this flavorful journey as we explore further than the delightful world of berries and embrace their potential to enhance our health and well-being.

Sources:

1. Basu, Arpita, and Timothy J. Strawbridge. "Oxidative Stress in Diabetes: The Role of Antioxidants and Pro-Oxidants." Antioxidants & Redox Signaling, vol. 7, no. 11-12, 2005, pp. 1608-19.
2. Seeram, Navindra P., et al. "Berries and Their Bioactive Compounds: Cardiovascular Benefits and Protective Mechanisms." Nutritional Neuroscience, vol. 7, no. 5-6, 2004, pp. 251-9.
3. McAnulty, Steven R., et al. "Effect of Blueberry Ingestion on Natural Killer Cell Counts, Oxidative Stress, and Inflammation Prior to and After 2.5 h of Running." Applied Physiology, Nutrition, and Metabolism, vol. 32, no. 6, 2007, pp. 133-7.
4. Stoner, Gary D. "Anthocyanins and Cancer Prevention." Proceedings of the Society for Experimental Biology and Medicine, vol. 218, no. 1, 1998, pp. 140-3.
5. Joseph, James A., et al. "Berries: Anti-Inflammatory Effects in Humans." The Journal of Agricultural and Food Chemistry, vol. 56, no. 3, 2008, pp. 922-7.

Chapter 13: Pineapple & Papaya: Tropical Fruits for Inflammation Relief

Amidst the lush landscapes of tropical paradises, two fruits stand out as vibrant symbols of sunshine and serenity: pineapple and papaya. These exotic treasures not only tantalize the taste buds with their sweet flavors and juicy textures but also offer powerful relief from inflammation, making them invaluable allies in the quest for optimal health and vitality.

At the heart of pineapple and papaya's healing power lies their rich array of enzymes, vitamins, and antioxidants. Pineapple boasts **bromelain**, a powerful enzyme renowned for its anti-inflammatory properties, while papaya contains **papain**, a proteolytic enzyme with similar benefits. *Together, these enzymes work to reduce swelling, soothe sore muscles, and promote healing throughout the body.*

But the benefits of pineapple and papaya extend far beyond their anti-inflammatory effects. These tropical fruits are also rich in vitamins A, C, and E, as well as an array of minerals and phytonutrients. Their potent antioxidant content helps to neutralize free radicals, reduce oxidative stress, and support overall immune function, making them essential components of a healthy diet.

But perhaps most notably, pineapple and papaya possess a unique ability to invigorate the senses and transport us to sun-kissed shores with every bite. Their sweet, juicy flesh and tropical flavors evoke feelings of joy and relaxation, making them a beloved addition to any meal or snack.

But how can we incorporate the healing power of pineapple and papaya into our daily lives? The possibilities are endless. From refreshing fruit salads and smoothie bowls to savory salsas and grilled kebabs, there are countless ways to enjoy the benefits of these tropical fruits. Whether eaten on their own or paired with other ingredients, pineapple and papaya add a burst of flavor and a touch of exoticism to every dish.

But a word of caution: while pineapple and papaya are generally safe for most people when consumed in moderation, some individuals may experience digestive discomfort or allergic reactions. As with any food or herbal remedy, it's important to listen to your body and consume these fruits as part of a balanced diet.

From mouthwatering recipes and refreshing beverages to nourishing skincare remedies, you'll discover a wealth of ways to harness the healing power of these tropical treasures. Join me on this flavorful journey as we explore more anti-inflammatory naturals beyond the sunny world of pineapple and papaya and embrace their potential to enhance our health and well-being.

Sources:

1. Hale, Laura P., et al. "Pineapple Bromelain Induces Autophagy, Facilitating Bacterial Clearance and Modulating Inflammation." Autophagy, vol. 10, no. 2, 2014, pp. 270-8.
2. Muhammad, Naveed, et al. "Bromelain: An Overview of Industrial Application and Purification Strategies." Critical Reviews in Food Science and Nutrition, vol. 56, no. 1, 2016, pp. 33-44.
3. Pandey, Kanti Bhooshan, and Syed Ibrahim Rizvi. "Plant Polyphenols as Dietary Antioxidants in Human Health and Disease." Oxidative Medicine and Cellular Longevity, vol. 2, no. 5, 2009, pp. 270-8.
4. Oliveira, Lívia Viganó de, et al. "Papain-Like Proteinases from Carica Papaya: Roles in the Regulation of Endogenous Proteins." Brazilian Journal of Pharmacognosy, vol. 23, no. 6, 2013, pp. 840-8.
5. Otsuki, Noriko, et al. "Papaya Seed Represents a Rich Source of Biologically Active Isothiocyanate." Journal of Agricultural and Food Chemistry, vol. 54, no. 10, 2006, pp. 3738-42.

Chapter 14: Broccoli Sprouts: Tiny Greens, Mighty Anti-Inflammatory

In the realm of superfoods, broccoli sprouts stand out as humble yet mighty warriors against inflammation. These tiny greens, bursting with vitality and brimming with health benefits, pack a powerful punch when it comes to soothing inflammation and promoting overall well-being. With their rich array of nutrients and bioactive compounds, broccoli sprouts offer a simple and effective way to harness the healing power of nature.

At the heart of broccoli sprouts' healing power lies their potent concentration of **sulforaphane**, a powerful antioxidant and anti-inflammatory compound. *Sulforaphane works by activating the body's natural defense mechanisms, scavenging harmful free radicals, and reducing inflammation at the cellular level. By targeting the root causes of inflammation, broccoli sprouts help to ease joint pain, reduce swelling, and support overall immune function.*

But the benefits of broccoli sprouts extend far beyond their anti-inflammatory effects. These tiny greens are also rich in vitamins, minerals, and phytonutrients, including vitamin C, vitamin K, and folate. Their potent antioxidant content helps to protect against cellular damage, boost immune function, and support detoxification pathways, making them an invaluable addition to any healthy diet.

But perhaps most notably, broccoli sprouts possess a unique ability to promote overall health and vitality with every bite. Whether added to salads, sandwiches, or smoothies, these crunchy greens add a burst of flavor and a dose of wellness to any meal. Their fresh, vibrant taste and crisp texture make them a versatile and delicious addition to a wide range of dishes.

How can we incorporate the healing power of broccoli sprouts into our daily lives? The possibilities are endless. From simple salads and sandwiches to hearty soups and stir-fries, there are countless ways to enjoy the benefits of broccoli sprouts. Whether eaten raw or lightly cooked, broccoli sprouts offer a convenient and delicious way to boost your intake of essential nutrients and support overall health and well-being.

But a word of caution: while broccoli sprouts are generally safe for most people when consumed in moderation, some individuals may experience digestive discomfort or allergic reactions. As with any food or herbal remedy, it's important to listen to your body and consume broccoli sprouts as part of a balanced diet.

By digging further, from mouthwatering recipes and refreshing beverages to nourishing skincare remedies, you can discover a wealth of ways to harness the healing power of these tiny greens. Join me as we explore more solutions than the remarkable world of broccoli sprouts and embrace their potential to enhance our health and well-being.

Sources:

1. Fahey, Jed W., et al. "Broccoli Sprouts: An Exceptionally Rich Source of Inducers of Enzymes That Protect Against Chemical Carcinogens." Proceedings of the National Academy of Sciences of the United States of America, vol. 94, no. 19, 1997, pp. 10367-72.

2. Angeloni, Cristina, et al. "Bioavailability of Sulforaphane from Broccoli Sprouts in Presence of Human Myrosinase as Determined by Measurement of Urinary Excretion of Sulforaphane Metabolites." Molecular Nutrition & Food Research, vol. 57, no. 11, 2013, pp. 2017-21.

3. Heber, David, et al. "Broccoli Sprouts: An Exceptionally Rich Source of Indolylmethylglucosinolates and Their Bioactive Products with Potential Health Benefits." Phytochemistry, vol. 65, no. 7, 2004, pp. 769-77.

4. Atwell, Lauren L., et al. "Evaluation of Cruciferous Vegetables for Anti-inflammatory Potential." Food Chemistry, vol. 138, no. 2-3, 2013, pp. 1156-62.

5. Lee, Jiyeon, et al. "Chemopreventive and Chemotherapeutic Effects of Intravesical Broccoli Sprout Extracts on Bladder Cancer Development." Journal of Cancer Prevention, vol. 19, no. 1, 2014, pp. 37-42.

Chapter 15: Cherries: Nature's Red Gems for Inflammation

In the orchards of nature's bounty, cherries stand out as vibrant red gems, enticing us with their sweet flavor and juicy texture. But beyond their delectable taste and aesthetic appeal, cherries harbor a remarkable secret: they are potent allies in the fight against inflammation. With their rich array of antioxidants and anti-inflammatory compounds, cherries offer a delicious and effective way to soothe inflammation and promote overall well-being.

At the heart of cherries' healing power lies their abundance of anthocyanins, flavonoids, and phenolic compounds. These potent antioxidants work synergistically to neutralize free radicals, reduce oxidative stress, and quell the flames of inflammation throughout the body. By targeting the root causes of inflammation, cherries help to ease joint pain, reduce muscle soreness, and support overall immune function.

But cherries' benefits extend far beyond their anti-inflammatory effects. Studies have shown that regular consumption of cherries may also help improve sleep quality, support heart health, and enhance athletic performance. Their ability to promote relaxation, reduce blood pressure, and increase endurance makes them a true superfood for both body and mind.

Perhaps most notably, cherries possess a unique ability to delight the senses and nourish the soul with every bite. Whether enjoyed fresh, dried, or juiced, cherries offer a burst of sweetness and a hint of tartness that tantalizes the taste buds and uplifts the spirit. Their vibrant color and succulent texture make them a beloved addition to any meal or snack.

How can we incorporate the healing power of cherries into our daily lives? The possibilities are endless. From refreshing salads and smoothies to decadent desserts and savory sauces, there are countless ways to enjoy the benefits of cherries. Whether eaten on their own or paired with other ingredients, cherries add a burst of flavor and a touch of elegance to every dish.

While cherries are generally safe for most people when consumed in moderation, some individuals may experience digestive discomfort or allergic reactions. As with any food or herbal remedy, it's important to listen to your body and consume cherries as part of a balanced diet.

Go ahead and explore the myriad ways in which cherries can be used to combat inflammation and promote overall health and vitality. From mouthwatering recipes and refreshing beverages to nourishing skincare remedies, you'll discover a wealth of ways to harness the healing power of these nature's red gems. Join me on this flavorful journey as we explore far beyond the delightful world of cherries and embrace their potential to enhance our health and well-being.

Sources:

1. Kelley, Darshan S., et al. "Sweet Bing Cherries Lower Circulating Concentrations of Markers for Chronic Inflammatory Diseases in Healthy Humans." The Journal of Nutrition, vol. 136, no. 4, 2006, pp. 981-6.
2. Kelley, Darshan S., et al. "Consumption of Bing Sweet Cherries Lowers Circulating Concentrations of Inflammation Markers in Healthy Men and Women." The FASEB Journal, vol. 20, no. 5, 2006, pp. A990-A991.
3. Jacob, Richard A., et al. "Consumption of Cherries Lowers Plasma Urate in Healthy Women." The Journal of Nutrition, vol. 133, no. 6, 2003, pp. 1826-9.
4. Seymour, E. Mitchell, et al. "Cherry Juice Proanthocyanidin Derivatives: Antioxidant and Cyclooxygenase Inhibitory Effects." Journal of Agricultural and Food Chemistry, vol. 52, no. 2, 2004, pp. 2659-64.
5. Connolly, Deborah A., et al. "Effects of Montmorency Tart Cherry (Prunus Cerasus L.) Consumption on Vascular Function in Men with Early Hypertension." American Journal of Clinical Nutrition, vol. 103, no. 6, 2016, pp. 1531-9.

Chapter 16: Flaxseeds: Tiny Seeds, Big Inflammation Benefits

Flaxseeds stand out as tiny powerhouses of goodness, offering a wealth of health benefits in their small, unassuming form. These humble seeds, derived from the flax plant, have been cherished for centuries for their remarkable nutritional profile and medicinal properties. Among their many virtues, flaxseeds are renowned for their ability to combat inflammation, making them a valuable addition to any diet seeking to promote overall well-being.

At the heart of flaxseeds' inflammation-fighting prowess lies their rich content of omega-3 fatty acids, particularly alpha-linolenic acid (ALA). These essential fatty acids play a crucial role in modulating the body's inflammatory response, helping to reduce inflammation at the cellular level. By inhibiting the production of pro-inflammatory molecules and promoting the synthesis of anti-inflammatory compounds, flaxseeds help to soothe inflammation and support overall immune function.

But the benefits of flaxseeds extend far beyond their anti-inflammatory effects. These tiny seeds are also rich in **lignans**, a type of phytoestrogen with powerful antioxidant properties. *Lignans help to neutralize free radicals, reduce oxidative stress, and protect against* *cellular damage, making them invaluable in promoting overall health and vitality.*

But perhaps most notably, flaxseeds possess a unique ability to support digestive health and promote regularity. Rich in soluble and insoluble fiber, flaxseeds help to promote bowel regularity, prevent constipation, and support a healthy gut microbiome. Their mucilaginous properties also help to soothe the digestive tract and alleviate symptoms of gastrointestinal discomfort.

How can we incorporate the healing power of flaxseeds into our daily lives? The possibilities are endless. From sprinkling ground flaxseeds on oatmeal or yogurt to adding whole flaxseeds to smoothies or baked goods, there are countless ways to enjoy the benefits of these versatile seeds. Whether eaten raw, toasted, or ground into meal, flaxseeds offer a convenient and delicious way to boost your intake of essential nutrients and support overall health and well-being.

While flaxseeds are generally safe for most people when consumed in moderation, some individuals may experience digestive discomfort or allergic reactions. As with any food or herbal remedy, it's important to listen to your body and consume flaxseeds as part of a balanced diet.

In the chapters that follow, we will explore beyond the myriad ways in which flaxseeds can be used to combat inflammation and promote overall health and vitality. Join me on this journey as we embrace the potential to enhance our health and well-being.

Sources:

1. Barceló-Coblijn, G., and R. Murphy. "Alpha-Linolenic Acid and Its Conversion to Longer Chain N-3 Fatty Acids: Benefits for Human Health and a Role in Maintaining Tissue n-3 Fatty Acid Levels." Progress in Lipid Research, vol. 48, no. 6, 2009, pp. 355-74.

2. Fukumitsu, Shinya, et al. "Flaxseed Lignan Attenuates High-Fat Diet-Induced Fat Accumulation and Induces Adiponectin Expression in Mice." British Journal of Nutrition, vol. 101, no. 11, 2009, pp. 1691-9.

3. Bloedon, L. T., et al. "Flaxseed and Cardiovascular Risk Factors: Results from a Double Blind, Randomized, Controlled Clinical Trial." Journal of the American College of Nutrition, vol. 27, no. 1, 2008, pp. 65-74.

4. Goyal, Ankit, et al. "Flax and Flaxseed Oil: An Ancient Medicine & Modern Functional Food." Journal of Food Science and Technology, vol. 51, no. 9, 2014, pp. 1633-53.

5. Hall, Christopher, et al. "Flaxseed." Advances in Nutrition, vol. 7, no. 4, 2016, pp. 759-61.

Chapter 17: Omega-3 Fatty Acids: Essential Oils for Inflammation

In the intricate tapestry of human health, few nutrients hold as much promise and potential as omega-3 fatty acids. These essential oils, found abundantly in certain **fish, nuts, and seeds**, play a pivotal role in modulating the body's inflammatory response and promoting overall well-being. With their remarkable anti-inflammatory properties, omega-3 fatty acids offer a natural and effective way to soothe inflammation and support optimal health.

At the heart of omega-3 fatty acids' inflammation-fighting prowess lies their unique chemical structure, which includes **eicosapentaenoic acid (EPA) and docosahexaenoic acid (DHA)**. These long-chain fatty acids are known for their ability to inhibit the production of pro-inflammatory molecules and promote the synthesis of anti-inflammatory compounds. *By modulating the balance of inflammatory mediators in the body, omega-3 fatty acids help to reduce inflammation at the cellular level, easing pain and promoting healing.*

But the benefits of omega-3 fatty acids extend far beyond their anti-inflammatory effects. These essential oils are also crucial for brain health, cardiovascular function, and immune support. Studies have shown that regular consumption of omega-3 fatty acids may help improve cognitive function, reduce the risk of heart disease, and enhance overall immune function, making them an indispensable part of a healthy diet.

But perhaps most notably, omega-3 fatty acids possess a unique ability to promote overall well-being and vitality with every dose. Whether obtained from fatty fish like salmon and mackerel or from plant-based sources like flaxseeds and walnuts, omega-3 fatty acids offer a simple and effective way to support overall health and vitality.

But how can we incorporate the healing power of omega-3 fatty acids into our daily lives? The possibilities are endless. From enjoying fatty fish as part of a balanced diet to supplementing with high-quality fish oil or algae oil capsules, there are countless ways to boost your intake of these essential nutrients. Whether eaten whole, cooked, or taken as a supplement, omega-3 fatty acids offer a convenient and delicious way to support optimal health and well-being.

But a word of caution: while omega-3 fatty acids are generally safe for most people when consumed in moderation, some individuals may experience digestive discomfort or allergic reactions. As with any dietary supplement, it's important to consult with a healthcare professional before beginning a regimen of omega-3 fatty acid supplementation, especially if you have underlying health conditions or are taking medications.

In the chapters that follow, we will explore the myriad ways in which omega-3 fatty acids can be used to combat inflammation and promote overall health and vitality. From mouthwatering recipes and nutritional supplements to nourishing skincare remedies, you'll discover a wealth of ways to harness the healing power of these essential oils. Join me on this journey as we explore the remarkable world of omega-3 fatty acids and embrace their potential to enhance our health and well-being.

Sources:

1. Calder, Philip C. "Omega-3 Fatty Acids and Inflammatory Processes: From Molecules to Man." Biochemical Society Transactions, vol. 45, no. 5, 2017, pp. 1105-15.
2. Serhan, Charles N. "Omega-3 Fatty Acids Are Pro-Resolving Mediators and Regulators of Inflammation." Lipids, vol. 43, no. 12, 2008, pp. 1123-7.
3. Calder, Philip C. "Omega-3 Polyunsaturated Fatty Acids and Inflammatory Processes: Nutrition or Pharmacology?" British Journal of Clinical Pharmacology, vol. 75, no. 3, 2013, pp. 645-62.
4. Simopoulos, Artemis P. "Omega-3 Fatty Acids in Inflammation and Autoimmune Diseases." Journal of the American College of Nutrition, vol. 21, no. 6, 2002, pp. 495-505.
5. Mozaffarian, Dariush, and Eric B. Rimm. "Fish Intake, Contaminants, and Human Health: Evaluating the Risks and the Benefits." JAMA, vol. 296, no. 15, 2006, pp. 1885-99.

Chapter 18: Magnesium: Mineral Magic for Inflammation Relief

In the intricate dance of biochemical processes within the human body, few minerals play as crucial a role as magnesium. Often referred to as the "mighty mineral," magnesium is involved in over 300 enzymatic reactions, including those that regulate inflammation. With its remarkable ability to soothe inflammation and promote overall well-being, magnesium emerges as a potent ally in the quest for optimal health.

At the heart of magnesium's inflammation-fighting prowess lies its role in modulating the body's inflammatory response. Magnesium helps to regulate the activity of inflammatory molecules, such as **cytokines and C-reactive protein**, thereby dampening the inflammatory cascade. *By promoting balance within the immune system, magnesium helps to reduce inflammation at the cellular level, easing discomfort and promoting healing.*

But the benefits of magnesium extend far beyond its anti-inflammatory effects. This essential mineral is also crucial for muscle function, nerve transmission, and bone health. Studies have shown that magnesium may help alleviate muscle cramps, improve sleep quality, and support cardiovascular function, making it an indispensable part of a healthy lifestyle.

But perpaps most notably, magnesium possesses a unique ability to promote relaxation and stress relief. As a natural muscle relaxant and nervine tonic, magnesium helps to calm the nervous system, reduce tension, and promote a sense of well-being. Its ability to ease anxiety, promote restful sleep, and enhance mood makes it a valuable tool for managing the stressors of modern life.

How can we ensure an adequate intake of magnesium in our daily lives? The answer lies in a balanced diet rich in magnesium-rich foods, such as leafy greens, nuts, seeds, and whole grains. Additionally, supplementation may be beneficial for individuals with inadequate dietary intake or increased magnesium needs due to factors such as stress, exercise, or certain medical conditions.

While magnesium is generally safe for most people when consumed in moderation, excessive intake may cause digestive upset or other adverse effects. As with any dietary supplement, it's important to consult with a healthcare professional before beginning a regimen of magnesium supplementation, especially if you have underlying health conditions or are taking medications.

From dietary sources and nutritional supplements to topical applications and therapeutic treatments, you'll discover a wealth of ways to harness the healing power of this mighty mineral. But join me as we explore the remarkable world far beyond magnesium and embrace its potential to enhance our health and well-being.

Sources:

1. Nielsen, Forrest H. "Magnesium Deficiency and Increased Inflammation: Current Perspectives." Journal of Inflammation Research, vol. 11, 2018, pp. 25-34.
2. De Baaij, Jeroen H.F., et al. "Magnesium in Man: Implications for Health and Disease." Physiological Reviews, vol. 95, no. 1, 2015, pp. 1-46.
3. Guerrero-Romero, Fernando, et al. "Oral Magnesium Supplementation Improves Insulin Sensitivity and Metabolic Control in Type 2 Diabetic Subjects: A Randomized Double-Blind Controlled Trial." Diabetes Care, vol. 28, no. 5, 2005, pp. 1147-52.
4. Nielsen, Forrest H. "Dietary Magnesium and Chronic Disease." Advances in Chronic Kidney Disease, vol. 25, no. 3, 2018, pp. 230-5.
5. Rosanoff, Andrea, et al. "Suboptimal Magnesium Status in the United States: Are the Health Consequences Underestimated?" Nutrition Reviews, vol. 70, no. 3, 2012, pp. 153-64.

Chapter 19: Avocado: Creamy Goodness, Anti-Inflammatory Properties

In the realm of nutrition, few fruits command as much attention and admiration as the avocado. With its rich, creamy texture and luscious flavor, the avocado is not only a culinary delight but also a nutritional powerhouse. Among its many virtues, the avocado boasts impressive anti-inflammatory properties, making it a valuable addition to any diet aimed at promoting overall health and well-being.

At the heart of the avocado's inflammation-fighting prowess lies its abundance of monounsaturated fats, particularly **oleic acid**. These healthy fats help to reduce inflammation at the cellular level by modulating the activity of inflammatory molecules and pathways. *By promoting balance within the immune system, avocados help to soothe inflammation, ease discomfort, and support overall immune function.*

The benefits of avocados extend far beyond their anti-inflammatory effects. These creamy fruits are also rich in fiber, vitamins, and minerals, including potassium, vitamin E, and folate. Their potent antioxidant content helps to neutralize free radicals, reduce oxidative stress, and protect against cellular damage, making them invaluable in promoting overall health and vitality.

Perhaps most notably, avocados possess a unique ability to promote satiety and stabilize blood sugar levels. Rich in fiber and healthy fats, avocados help to slow digestion, regulate appetite, and prevent spikes and crashes in blood sugar. Their ability to promote feelings of fullness and satisfaction makes them a valuable ally in the quest for healthy weight management and metabolic balance.

So how can we incorporate the healing power of avocados into our daily lives? The possibilities are endless. From simple avocado toast and guacamole to creamy smoothies and salad dressings, there are countless ways to enjoy the benefits of avocados. Whether eaten on their own or paired with other ingredients, avocados add a luxurious texture and a wealth of nutrients to any dish.

But a word of caution: while avocados are generally safe for most people when consumed in moderation, some individuals may experience digestive discomfort or allergic reactions. As with any food or herbal remedy, it's important to listen to your body and consume avocados as part of a balanced diet.

From mouthwatering recipes and nutritious snacks to nourishing skincare remedies, there exists a wealth of ways to harness the healing power of these creamy fruits. Remain with me as we explore other herbs in addition to the delightful world of avocados and as we embrace their potential to enhance our health and well-being.

Sources:

1. Dreher, Mark L., and Adrienne J. Davenport. "Hass Avocado Composition and Potential Health Effects." Critical Reviews in Food Science and Nutrition, vol. 53, no. 7, 2013, pp. 738-50.
2. Wien, Michelle, et al. "A Randomized 3x3 Crossover Study to Evaluate the Effect of Hass Avocado Intake on Post-Ingestive Satiety, Glucose and Insulin Levels, and Subsequent Energy Intake in Overweight Adults." Nutrition Journal, vol. 12, no. 1, 2013, pp. 155.
3. Fulgoni, Victor L., et al. "Avocado Consumption Is Associated with Better Diet Quality and Nutrient Intake, and Lower Metabolic Syndrome Risk in US Adults: Results from the National Health and Nutrition Examination Survey (NHANES) 2001-2008." Nutrition Journal, vol. 12, no. 1, 2013, pp. 1-9.
4. Basu, Arpita, et al. "Berries: Emerging Impact on Cardiovascular Health." Nutrition Reviews, vol. 68, no. 3, 2010, pp. 168-77.
5. Guasch-Ferré, Marta, et al. "Frequency of Nut Consumption and Mortality Risk in the PREDIMED Nutrition Intervention Trial." BMC Medicine, vol. 11, no. 1, 2013, pp. 1-11.

Chapter 20: Nettle Leaf: Sting with Soothing Powers

In the verdant corners of nature, nestled among the foliage, hides a plant with a sting and a secret: the nettle leaf. Despite its prickly reputation, nettle leaf harbors remarkable soothing powers, making it a cherished ally in the quest for natural inflammation relief. With its rich history in herbal medicine and its potent anti-inflammatory properties, nettle leaf emerges as a formidable force in promoting overall health and well-being.

At the heart of nettle leaf's healing prowess lies its impressive array of bioactive compounds, including **flavonoids, phenolic acids, and polysaccharides.** These plant-based chemicals work synergistically to reduce inflammation, inhibit allergic responses, and promote tissue repair. *By modulating the body's inflammatory pathways, nettle leaf helps to soothe discomfort, ease swelling, and support overall immune function.*

The benefits of nettle leaf extend far beyond its anti-inflammatory effects. This versatile herb is also rich in vitamins, minerals, and antioxidants, including vitamin C, vitamin K, and iron. Its potent antioxidant content helps to neutralize free radicals, reduce oxidative stress, and protect against cellular damage, making it invaluable for overall health and vitality.

Most notably, nettle leaf possesses a unique ability to support respiratory health and alleviate allergy symptoms. Studies have shown that nettle leaf may help reduce hay fever symptoms, improve allergic rhinitis, and support lung function. Its natural antihistamine properties help to relieve nasal congestion, sneezing, and itching, making it a valuable tool for seasonal allergy relief.

In what ways can we harness the healing power of nettle leaf in our daily lives? The possibilities are endless. From brewing nourishing herbal teas and infusions to incorporating dried nettle leaf into soups, stews, and stir-fries, there are countless ways to enjoy the benefits of this versatile herb. Whether consumed as a tea, tincture, or capsule, nettle leaf offers a convenient and effective way to support overall health and well-being.

Even though nettle leaf is generally safe for most people when consumed in moderation, some individuals may experience allergic reactions or digestive discomfort. As with any herbal remedy, it's important to consult with a healthcare professional before beginning a regimen of nettle leaf supplementation, especially if you have underlying health conditions or are taking medications.

From traditional remedies and herbal preparations to innovative culinary creations and skincare solutions, there are a wealth of ways to harness the healing power of this prickly yet potent herb. Proceed onward with me as we explore other herbs apart from this remarkable world of nettle leaf.

Sources:

1. Roschek Jr, Bill, et al. "Nettle Extract (Urtica Dioica) Affects Key Receptors and Enzymes Associated with Allergic Rhinitis." Phytotherapy Research, vol. 23, no. 7, 2009, pp. 920-6.

2. Mittman, Paul. "Randomized, Double-Blind Study of Freeze-Dried Urtica Dioica in the Treatment of Allergic Rhinitis." Planta Medica, vol. 56, no. 1, 1990, pp. 44-7.

3. Hajhashemi, Valiollah, et al. "Antihistaminic and Anticholinergic Activity of Urtica Dioica Leaf Extract in Isolated Rat Ileum." Medical Journal of the Islamic Republic of Iran, vol. 27, no. 3, 2013, pp. 141-8.

4. Schöttner, M., et al. "Lignans from the Roots of Urtica Dioica and Their Metabolites Bind to Human Sex Hormone Binding Globulin (SHBG)." Planta Medica, vol. 62, no. 6, 1996, pp. 529-32.

5. Sarrell, E. Michael, et al. "Treatment of Hay Fever with Allergen-Specific Cytokines." Archives of Otolaryngology-Head & Neck Surgery, vol. 129, no. 5, 2003, pp. 569-72.

Chapter 21: Licorice Root: Sweet Relief for Inflammation

In the rich tapestry of herbal medicine, licorice root emerges as a sweet and soothing remedy for inflammation. With its distinct flavor and potent medicinal properties, licorice root has been cherished for centuries as a natural remedy for a wide range of ailments. Among its many virtues, licorice root offers sweet relief for inflammation, making it a valuable ally in the quest for optimal health and well-being.

At the heart of licorice root's inflammation-fighting prowess lies its abundance of bioactive compounds, including **glycyrrhizin, flavonoids, and saponins**. These plant-based chemicals work synergistically to reduce inflammation, soothe irritation, and promote tissue repair. *By modulating the body's inflammatory pathways, licorice root helps to ease discomfort, support healing, and restore balance to the body.*

Licorice root is also renowned for its ability to support digestive health, promote respiratory function, and enhance immune response. Studies have shown that licorice root may help alleviate symptoms of gastrointestinal disorders, respiratory infections, and autoimmune conditions, making it a valuable tool for overall health and vitality.

A very important attribute that licorice root possesses is its unique ability to support adrenal function and alleviate stress. As an adaptogenic herb, licorice root helps to regulate the body's stress response, improve energy levels, and enhance resilience to stressors. Its natural cortisol-like effects help to promote a sense of calm, balance, and well-being, making it a valuable ally in managing the demands of modern life.

But how can we incorporate the healing power of licorice root into our daily lives? The possibilities are endless. From brewing soothing herbal teas and decoctions to adding licorice root extract to culinary creations and skincare formulations, there are countless ways to enjoy the benefits of this versatile herb. Whether consumed internally or applied topically, licorice root offers a convenient and effective way to support overall health and well-being.

Licorice root is generally safe for most people when consumed in moderation, but excessive intake may cause adverse effects, especially in individuals with certain health conditions or medications. So, as with any herbal remedy, it's important to consult with a healthcare professional before beginning a regimen of licorice root supplementation, especially if you have underlying health conditions or are pregnant or breastfeeding.

From traditional remedies and herbal preparations to innovative culinary creations and skincare solutions, you'll discover a wealth of ways to harness the healing power of this sweet and soothing herb. But join me on this journey as we explore more than the remarkable world of licorice root in the following chapters.

Sources:

1. Fiore, Cristina, et al. "Antiviral Effects of Glycyrrhiza Species." Phytotherapy Research, vol. 22, no. 2, 2008, pp. 141-8.

2. Fiore, Cristina, et al. "A Review of Pharmacological Activities of Glycyrrhiza Glabra L. and Its Bioactive Compounds." Phytotherapy Research, vol. 28, no. 7, 2014, pp. 949-69.

3. Wang, Chen-Ting, et al. "Glycyrrhizic Acid Alleviates 2,4,6-Trinitrobenzene Sulfonic Acid-Induced Colitis in Mice via Reducing Inflammation and Repairing Epithelium." Frontiers in Pharmacology, vol. 11, 2020, pp. 1-11.

4. Armanini, Decio, et al. "Treatment of Polycystic Ovary Syndrome with Spironolactone Plus Licorice." European Journal of Obstetrics & Gynecology and Reproductive Biology, vol. 131, no. 1, 2007, pp. 61-7.

5. Wittschier, Nina, et al. "Aqueous Extracts and Polysaccharides from Liquorice Roots (Glycyrrhiza Glabra L.) Inhibit Adhesion of Helicobacter Pylori to Human Gastric Mucosa." Journal of Ethnopharmacology, vol. 125, no. 2, 2009, pp. 218-23.

Chapter 22: Echinacea: Immune-Boosting Herb, Inflammation Soother

In the realm of herbal medicine, few plants command as much respect and admiration as Echinacea. With its vibrant petals and potent medicinal properties, Echinacea stands as a symbol of vitality and resilience. Among its many virtues, Echinacea shines as an immune-boosting herb and inflammation soother, offering a natural solution to promote overall health and well-being.

At the heart of Echinacea's healing prowess lies its rich array of bioactive compounds, including **alkamides, polysaccharides, and flavonoids**. These plant-based chemicals work synergistically to support immune function, enhance white blood cell activity, and reduce inflammation. *By modulating the body's immune response, Echinacea helps to defend against infections, soothe inflammation, and promote healing.*

The benefits of Echinacea extend far beyond its immune-boosting effects. This versatile herb is also renowned for its ability to support respiratory health, alleviate cold and flu symptoms, and promote overall wellness. Studies have shown that Echinacea may help reduce the severity and duration of respiratory infections, alleviate symptoms such as cough and congestion, and support immune resilience, making it a valuable ally in the fight against seasonal illness.

Most notably, Echinacea possesses a unique ability to promote tissue repair and wound healing. Its anti-inflammatory and antimicrobial properties help to soothe irritation, reduce swelling, and protect against infection, making it invaluable for promoting overall skin health and vitality. Whether applied topically or taken internally, Echinacea offers a convenient and effective way to support overall well-being.

But how can we harness the healing power of Echinacea in our daily lives? The possibilities are endless. From brewing immune-boosting herbal teas and tinctures to incorporating Echinacea extract into skincare formulations and throat lozenges, there are countless ways to enjoy the benefits of this versatile herb. Whether used preventatively during cold and flu season or as a natural remedy to soothe inflammation and promote healing, Echinacea offers a valuable tool for supporting overall health and vitality.

But a word of caution: while Echinacea is generally safe for most people when consumed in moderation, some individuals may experience allergic reactions or digestive discomfort. As with any herbal remedy, it's important to consult with a healthcare professional before beginning a regimen of Echinacea supplementation, especially if you have underlying health conditions or are pregnant or breastfeeding.

In the chapters that follow, we will go beyond the myriad ways in which Echinacea can be used to support immune health, soothe inflammation, and promote overall well-being. From traditional remedies and herbal preparations to innovative skincare solutions and immune-boosting recipes, you'll discover a wealth of more ways to harness the healing power of natural anti-inflammatories.

Sources:

1. Hudson, James B. "Applications of the Phytomedicine Echinacea Purpurea (Purple Coneflower) in Infectious Diseases." Journal of Biomedicine and Biotechnology, vol. 2012, 2012, pp. 1-16.

2. Pleschka, Stephan. "Anti-Viral Properties and Mode of Action of Standardized Echinacea Purpurea Extract Against Highly Pathogenic Avian Influenza Virus (H5N1, H7N7) and Swine-Origin H1N1 (S-OIV)." Virology Journal, vol. 6, no. 1, 2009, pp. 1-12.

3. Barrett, Bruce, et al. "Treatment of the Common Cold with Unrefined Echinacea: A Randomized, Double-Blind, Placebo-Controlled Trial." Annals of Internal Medicine, vol. 137, no. 12, 2002, pp. 939-46.

4. Sharma, Manju, et al. "Inhibition of UVA and UVB Induced Oxidative Stress and Premature Senescence in Human Skin Fibroblasts by Echinacea Aerial Parts Extract." Journal of Photochemistry and Photobiology B: Biology, vol. 153, 2015, pp. 347-55.

5. Ritchie, Mark R., et al. "Echinacea Species (Echinacea Angustifolia (DC.) Hell., Echinacea Pallida (Nutt.) Nutt., Echinacea Purpurea (L.) Moench): A Review of Their Chemistry, Pharmacology and Clinical Properties." Journal of Pharmacy and Pharmacology, vol. 58, no. 12, 2006, pp. 1537-49.

Chapter 23: Aloe Vera: Cooling Gel, Inflammation Relief

In the sun-kissed lands where desert meets shore, thrives a plant with a gift of healing: Aloe vera. Renowned for its cooling gel and potent medicinal properties, Aloe vera stands as an emblem of rejuvenation and restoration. Among its many virtues, Aloe vera offers soothing relief for inflammation, providing a natural remedy for promoting overall health and well-being.

At the heart of Aloe vera's healing prowess lies its succulent leaves, which contain a rich reservoir of bioactive compounds, including **polysaccharides, glycoproteins, and antioxidants**. These plant-based chemicals work synergistically to reduce inflammation, soothe irritation, and promote tissue repair. *By modulating the body's inflammatory pathways, Aloe vera helps to ease discomfort, support healing, and restore balance to the body.*

The benefits of Aloe vera extend far beyond its anti-inflammatory effects. This versatile plant is also renowned for its ability to promote skin health, alleviate sunburn, and enhance wound healing. Studies have shown that Aloe vera gel may help reduce redness, swelling, and pain associated with sunburn, promote collagen production, and accelerate the healing process, making it a valuable ally in maintaining healthy, radiant skin.

Aloe vera possesses a unique ability to hydrate and nourish the skin from within. Its natural humectant properties help to draw moisture to the skin, keeping it soft, supple, and hydrated. Whether applied topically as a soothing gel or consumed internally as a nutritional supplement, Aloe vera offers a convenient and effective way to support overall skin health and vitality.

Just how can we harness the healing power of Aloe vera in our daily lives? From applying fresh Aloe vera gel to sun-kissed skin to incorporating Aloe vera juice into smoothies and beverages, there are countless ways to enjoy the benefits of this versatile plant. Whether used topically or internally, Aloe vera offers a valuable tool for promoting overall health and well-being.

Aloe vera is generally safe for most people when used externally or consumed in moderation but some individuals may experience allergic reactions or digestive discomfort. So as with any herbal remedy, it's important to perform a patch test before applying Aloe vera gel to the skin and to consult with a healthcare professional before beginning a regimen of Aloe vera supplementation, especially if you have underlying health conditions or are pregnant or breastfeeding.

From traditional remedies and skincare formulations to innovative culinary creations and nutritional supplements, there is a wealth of ways to harness the healing power of this versatile plant. Join me on this journey as we go beyond the remarkable world of Aloe vera.

Sources:

1. Surjushe, Amar, et al. "Aloe Vera: A Short Review." Indian Journal of Dermatology, vol. 53, no. 4, 2008, pp. 163-6.

2. Maenthaisong, Ratree, et al. "The Efficacy of Aloe Vera Used for Burn Wound Healing: A Systematic Review." Burns, vol. 33, no. 6, 2007, pp. 713-8.

3. Tabassum, Nahida, and Mariya Hamdani. "Plants Used to Treat Skin Diseases." Pharmacognosy Reviews, vol. 7, no. 13, 2013, pp. 52-60.

4. Foster, Steven, and Rebecca L. Johnson. Desk Reference to Nature's Medicine. National Geographic, 2006.

5. Radha, Maharjan, and Elizabeth Olson. "Phytochemicals of Aloe Vera and Their Pharmacological Activities: A Review." Journal of Nepal Pharmaceutical Association, vol. 24, no. 1, 2011, pp. 62-8.

Chapter 24: Devil's Claw: Nature's Answer to Joint Inflammation

In the arid plains of Southern Africa, amidst the harsh terrain, thrives a plant with a powerful remedy hidden within its roots: Devil's Claw. Revered for centuries by indigenous peoples for its potent medicinal properties, Devil's Claw emerges as nature's answer to joint inflammation. With its unique blend of bioactive compounds, this botanical treasure offers a natural solution for promoting joint health and overall well-being.

At the heart of Devil's Claw's healing prowess lies its rich reservoir of **iridoid glycosides, harpagoside** being the most prominent. These compounds possess powerful anti-inflammatory properties, helping to reduce pain, swelling, and stiffness associated with joint inflammation. *By modulating the body's inflammatory pathways, Devil's Claw offers relief from discomfort, promoting greater mobility and flexibility.*

The benefits of Devil's Claw extend beyond its anti-inflammatory effects. This remarkable herb is also known for its analgesic properties, offering relief from the chronic pain often associated with conditions such as osteoarthritis and rheumatoid arthritis. Studies have shown that Devil's Claw may help to alleviate pain, improve joint function, and enhance quality of life for individuals living with these conditions.

Devil's Claw possesses a unique ability to support overall joint health and cartilage integrity. Its antioxidant properties help to protect against oxidative damage and promote tissue repair, while its anti-inflammatory effects help to reduce the degradation of cartilage and inhibit the progression of joint-related conditions. Whether used preventatively or as a complementary therapy, Devil's Claw offers hope for those seeking relief from joint inflammation.

How do we harness the healing power of Devil's Claw in our daily lives? The answer lies in a balanced approach that includes both internal and external applications. Devil's Claw supplements, available in various forms such as capsules, extracts, and teas, offer a convenient way to incorporate this botanical remedy into your daily routine. Additionally, topical preparations containing Devil's Claw extract can provide targeted relief for sore, achy joints.

Devil's Claw is generally safe for most people when used as directed, however some individuals may experience digestive upset or allergic reactions. As with any herbal remedy, it's important to consult with a healthcare professional before beginning a regimen of Devil's Claw supplementation, especially if you have underlying health conditions or are taking medications.

From traditional remedies and herbal preparations to innovative supplements and therapeutic treatments, you'll discover a wealth of ways to harness the healing power of this remarkable herb.

Sources:

1. Chrubasik, Sigrun, et al. "Harpagophytum Procumbens for Osteoarthritis and Low Back Pain: A Systematic Review." BMC Complementary and Alternative Medicine, vol. 2, no. 1, 2002, pp. 1-8.
2. Gagnier, Joel J., et al. "Devil's Claw (Harpagophytum Procumbens) as a Treatment for Osteoarthritis: A Review of Efficacy and Safety." Journal of Alternative and Complementary Medicine, vol. 16, no. 11, 2010, pp. 1169-78.
3. Akhtar, Nahida, et al. "Harpagophytum Procumbens: An Ethnopharmacological, Phytochemical and Pharmacological Review." Journal of Pharmacy and Pharmacology, vol. 69, no. 10, 2017, pp. 1379-93.
4. Wegener, Thomas, and Reinhard Lüpke. "Treatment of Patients with Arthrosis of Hip or Knee with an Aqueous Extract of Devil's Claw (Harpagophytum Procumbens DC.)." Phytotherapy Research, vol. 15, no. 4, 2001, pp. 344-50.
5. Chantre, Philippe, and François Cappelaere. "Efficacy and Tolerance of Harpagophytum Procumbens versus Diacerhein in Treatment of Osteoarthritis." Phytomedicine, vol. 11, no. 2-3, 2004, pp. 148-56.

Chapter 25: Reishi Mushroom: Fungus with Anti-Inflammatory Benefits

In the quiet depths of ancient forests, amidst the fallen leaves and moss-covered logs, thrives a remarkable fungus with a gift of healing: the Reishi mushroom. Revered for centuries in traditional Chinese medicine for its potent medicinal properties, Reishi emerges as a powerful ally in the fight against inflammation. With its unique blend of bioactive compounds, this mystical mushroom offers a natural solution for promoting overall health and well-being.

At the heart of Reishi's healing prowess lies its rich array of **polysaccharides, triterpenes, and antioxidants**. These potent compounds work synergistically to reduce inflammation, modulate immune function, and promote tissue repair. *By targeting inflammatory pathways within the body, Reishi helps to soothe discomfort, ease swelling, and support overall immune health.*

The benefits of Reishi extend far beyond its anti-inflammatory effects. This versatile mushroom is also revered for its adaptogenic properties, helping to promote resilience to stress, enhance energy levels, and support mental clarity. Studies have shown that Reishi may help reduce fatigue, improve sleep quality, and enhance overall vitality, making it a valuable ally in navigating the demands of modern life.

Most notably, Reishi possesses a unique ability to support cardiovascular health and promote longevity. Its antioxidant properties help to protect against oxidative stress and reduce the risk of chronic diseases such as heart disease and diabetes. By promoting circulation, lowering cholesterol levels, and supporting blood vessel health, Reishi offers comprehensive support for a healthy heart and circulatory system.

But how could we harness the healing power of Reishi in our daily lives? The answer lies in incorporating this remarkable mushroom into our daily routine. Reishi supplements, available in various forms such as capsules, extracts, and teas, offer a convenient way to enjoy the benefits of this potent fungus. Additionally, incorporating Reishi into culinary creations such as soups, stews, and teas allows us to savor its earthy flavor while reaping its many health benefits.

Caution: Reishi is generally safe for most people when consumed in moderation, but some individuals may experience digestive upset or allergic reactions. As with any herbal remedy, it's important to consult with a healthcare professional before beginning a regimen of Reishi supplementation, especially if you have underlying health conditions or are pregnant or breastfeeding.

From traditional remedies and herbal preparations to innovative supplements and culinary creations, you can discover a wealth of ways to harness the healing power of this remarkable mushroom. But join me on this journey as we go far and beyond the remarkable world of Reishi.

Sources:

1. Wasser, Solomon P., and Alexander L. Weis. "Therapeutic Effects of Substances Occurring in Higher Basidiomycetes Mushrooms: A Modern Perspective." Critical Reviews in Immunology, vol. 19, no. 1, 1999, pp. 65-96.

2. Lin, Zhi-bin, et al. "Ganoderma Lucidum Polysaccharides Attenuate Cisplatin-Induced Nephrotoxicity In Mice." Journal of Cellular and Molecular Medicine, vol. 18, no. 3, 2014, pp. 518-29.

3. Gao, Yi, et al. "Effects of Ganoderma Lucidum Polysaccharides on Chronic Pancreatitis and Intestinal Microbiota in Mice." International Journal of Biological Macromolecules, vol. 126, 2019, pp. 273-83.

4. Wang, Xia, et al. "Ganoderma Lucidum Polysaccharides Prevent Palmitic Acid-Evoked Apoptosis and Autophagy in Intestinal Porcine Epithelial Cells via Restoration of Mitochondrial Function and Regulation of JNK and AMPK/Akt/mTOR Signaling Pathways." Journal of Functional Foods, vol. 61, 2019, pp. 1-12.

5. Zhang, Jie, et al. "A Review of Ganoderma Lucidum Pharmacological Activity and Clinical Practice in Promoting Health." Proceedings of the Nutrition Society, vol. 75, no. 3, 2016, pp. 321-34.

Chapter 26: Oregano: Culinary Herb, Anti-Inflammatory Wonder

In the sun-drenched fields of the Mediterranean, amidst the fragrant herbs and olive groves, thrives a culinary gem with a secret: Oregano. Beyond its role as a flavorful seasoning, oregano emerges as an anti-inflammatory wonder, offering a potent remedy for promoting overall health and well-being. With its rich array of bioactive compounds, this humble herb packs a powerful punch against inflammation, making it a valuable addition to any kitchen pantry.

At the heart of oregano's healing prowess lies its abundance of volatile oils, including **carvacrol, thymol, and rosmarinic acid**. These potent compounds work synergistically to reduce inflammation, inhibit the production of inflammatory enzymes, and neutralize free radicals. *By targeting inflammatory pathways within the body, oregano helps to soothe discomfort, ease swelling, and support overall immune health.*

Oregano is also revered for its antimicrobial properties, helping to fight off harmful bacteria, viruses, and fungi. Studies have shown that oregano oil may help to combat infections, support gut health, and boost immune function, making it a valuable ally in maintaining overall wellness.

Most notably, oregano possesses a unique ability to support digestive health and promote optimal digestion. Its carminative properties help to relieve gas, bloating, and indigestion, while its antispasmodic effects help to soothe intestinal cramps and discomfort. Whether used fresh or dried, oregano offers a flavorful addition to culinary creations while supporting digestive wellness.

You may be wondering how we can harness the healing power of oregano in our daily lives. The answer lies in incorporating this versatile herb into our favorite recipes. Whether sprinkled over pizza, stirred into pasta sauce, or infused into salad dressings, oregano adds depth of flavor and nutritional value to a wide range of dishes. Additionally, oregano oil supplements offer a concentrated source of the herb's active compounds, providing targeted support for inflammation relief and immune health.

Inasmuchas oregano is generally safe for most people when used as a culinary herb, concentrated oregano oil supplements may cause digestive upset or allergic reactions in some individuals. As with any herbal remedy, it's important to consult with a healthcare professional before beginning a regimen of oregano supplementation, especially if you have underlying health conditions or are pregnant or breastfeeding.

From traditional remedies and culinary creations to innovative supplements and therapeutic treatments, you'll discover a wealth of ways that harness the healing power of this versatile herb. Continue alongside me as we explore the remarkable world of oregano and embrace its potential to enhance our health and vitality and venture much further and beyond.

Sources:

1. Force, Maria, et al. "Antimicrobial Activity of Essential Oils from Mediterranean Aromatic Plants Against Several Foodborne and Spoilage Bacteria." Food Science and Technology International, vol. 6, no. 9, 2000, pp. 815-21.
2. Li, Y., et al. "Inhibitory Effects of Carvacrol on LPS-Induced Inflammation in RAW264.7 Cells." Cellular and Molecular Biology, vol. 62, no. 3, 2016, pp. 60-4.
3. Maggio, Antonella, et al. "Essential Oils and Pure Volatile Compounds as Potential Drugs in Alzheimer's Disease Therapy: An Updated Review of the Literature." Current Pharmaceutical Design, vol. 23, no. 26, 2017, pp. 4005-16.
4. Sakkas, Hercules, et al. "Antibacterial Activity of Oregano Essential Oil Alone and in Combination with Antibiotics Against Extended-Spectrum β-Lactamase (ESBL)-Producing Escherichia Coli." Phytotherapy Research, vol. 31, no. 2, 2017, pp. 213-22.
5. Aprotosoaie, Ana Clara, et al. "Lycopene and Its Antioxidant Role in the Prevention of Cardiovascular Diseases—A Critical Review." Critical Reviews in Food Science and Nutrition, vol. 57, no. 6, 2017, pp. 1297-1309.

Chapter 27: Thyme: Fragrant Herb, Inflammation Fighter

In the sun-drenched hillsides of the Mediterranean, amidst the wildflowers and aromatic shrubs, flourishes a herbaceous marvel with a hidden strength: Thyme. Beyond its role as a culinary delight, thyme emerges as a formidable inflammation fighter, offering a potent remedy for promoting overall health and well-being. With its unique blend of bioactive compounds, this fragrant herb stands as a powerful ally in the quest for inflammation relief.

At the heart of thyme's healing prowess lies its rich concentration of essential oils, including **thymol, carvacrol, and linalool**. These potent compounds possess strong antioxidant and anti-inflammatory properties, helping to combat oxidative stress, reduce inflammation, and support overall immune function. *By modulating inflammatory pathways within the body, thyme offers relief from discomfort, promotes healing, and enhances well-being.*

Thyme is also revered for its antimicrobial properties, helping to fend off harmful bacteria, viruses, and fungi. Studies have shown that thyme essential oil may help combat infections, support respiratory health, and promote overall wellness, making it a valuable addition to any natural medicine cabinet.

Thyme also, most importantly, possesses a unique ability to *support respiratory health and soothe coughs and congestion.* Its expectorant properties help to *loosen mucus, clear airways, and ease breathing,* while its antispasmodic effects help to *reduce coughing fits and irritation.* Whether used in teas, tinctures, or steam inhalations, thyme offers a natural solution for respiratory discomfort and congestion.

But how can we harness the healing power of thyme in our daily lives? The answer lies in incorporating this fragrant herb into our culinary creations and natural remedies. Whether sprinkled over roasted vegetables, infused into herbal teas, or blended into homemade cough syrups, thyme adds depth of flavor and therapeutic benefits to a wide range of dishes and remedies. Additionally, thyme essential oil can be diffused aromatically or applied topically for added respiratory support and immune enhancement.

Altough thyme is generally safe for most people when used as a culinary herb or aromatherapy ingredient, concentrated thyme essential oil may cause skin irritation or allergic reactions in some individuals. As with any herbal remedy, it's important to perform a patch test before using thyme essential oil topically and to consult with a healthcare professional before beginning a regimen of thyme supplementation, especially if you have underlying health conditions or are pregnant or breastfeeding.

In the chapters that follow, we will explore the myriad ways in which thyme can be used to promote inflammation relief, support respiratory health, and enhance overall well-being. From traditional remedies and culinary creations to innovative supplements and aromatherapy treatments, you'll discover a wealth of ways to harness the healing power of this fragrant herb. Join me on this journey as we explore the remarkable world of thyme and embrace its potential to enhance our health and vitality.

Sources:

1. Gülçin, İlhami, et al. "Evaluation of the Antioxidant and Antimicrobial Activities of Clary Sage (Salvia Sclarea L.)." Turkish Journal of Agriculture and Forestry, vol. 34, no. 2, 2010, pp. 137-45.
2. De Martino, Laura, et al. "Chemical Composition and Antimicrobial Activity of Essential Oils from Aerial Parts of Salvia L. Species." Natural Product Communications, vol. 4, no. 7, 2009, pp. 1027-34.
3. Russo, Alessandra, et al. "Chemical Composition and Antimicrobial Activity of Essential Oils of Three Mediterranean Lamiaceae." Molecules, vol. 13, no. 2, 2008, pp. 461-70.
4. Knobloch, Karin, et al. "Antibacterial and Antifungal Properties of Essential Oil Components." Journal of Essential Oil Research, vol. 1, no. 3, 1989, pp. 119-28.
5. Siurin, Sergey A., et al. "Thymus Serpyllum L. Essential Oil: Chemical Composition and Antimicrobial Activity." Journal of Essential Oil Research, vol. 17, no. 6, 2005, pp. 681-3.

Chapter 28: Sage: Savory Herb, Soothing Inflammation

In the sun-kissed meadows and rocky slopes of the Mediterranean, a herb with a rich history and potent healing properties thrives: Sage. Beyond its culinary prowess and aromatic allure, sage emerges as a potent ally in the battle against inflammation. With its unique blend of bioactive compounds, this savory herb offers a natural remedy for promoting overall health and well-being.

At the heart of sage's healing prowess lies its abundance of **volatile oils, flavonoids, and phenolic acids**. These potent compounds work synergistically to reduce inflammation, neutralize free radicals, and promote tissue repair. *By targeting inflammatory pathways within the body, sage helps to soothe discomfort, ease swelling, and support overall immune function.*

But the benefits of sage extend far beyond its anti-inflammatory effects. This versatile herb is also revered for its antimicrobial properties, helping to fend off harmful bacteria, viruses, and fungi. Studies have shown that *sage essential oil may help combat infections, support oral health, and promote overall wellness*, making it a valuable addition to any natural medicine cabinet.

But perhaps most notably, sage possesses a unique ability to support cognitive function and enhance mental clarity. Its antioxidant properties help to protect against oxidative stress and neurodegeneration, while its cognitive-enhancing effects help to improve memory, focus, and mood. Whether used in teas, aromatherapy, or culinary creations, sage offers a natural solution for promoting brain health and vitality.

But how can we harness the healing power of sage in our daily lives? The answer lies in incorporating this versatile herb into our favorite recipes and natural remedies. Whether sprinkled over roasted vegetables, infused into herbal teas, or blended into homemade throat lozenges, sage adds depth of flavor and therapeutic benefits to a wide range of dishes and remedies. Additionally, sage essential oil can be diffused aromatically or applied topically for added immune support and cognitive enhancement.

But a word of caution: while sage is generally safe for most people when used as a culinary herb or aromatherapy ingredient, concentrated sage essential oil may cause skin irritation or allergic reactions in some individuals. As with any herbal remedy, it's important to perform a patch test before using sage essential oil topically and to consult with a healthcare professional before beginning a regimen of sage supplementation, especially if you have underlying health conditions or are pregnant or breastfeeding.

In the chapters that follow, we will explore the myriad other ways in addition to sage in which herbs can be used to promote inflammation relief, support cognitive function, and enhance overall well-being. From traditional remedies and culinary creations to innovative supplements and aromatherapy treatments, we'll discover a wealth of ways to harness the healing power of more herbs. Join me on this journey as we explore the remarkable world of herbs and embrace their potential to enhance our health and vitality.

Sources:

1. Perry, Nigel S.L., et al. "Essential Oils from Dalmatian Sage (Salvia Officinalis L.): Variations Among Individuals, Plant Parts, Seasons, and Sites." Journal of Agricultural and Food Chemistry, vol. 48, no. 6, 2000, pp. 2048-54.

2. De Martino, Laura, et al. "Chemical Composition and Antimicrobial Activity of Essential Oils from Aerial Parts of Salvia L. Species." Natural Product Communications, vol. 4, no. 7, 2009, pp. 1027-34.

3. Ghorbani, Ahmad, and Faraz Mohebati. "Sage, Salvia Officinalis, and Its Active Ingredients: A Review." Iranian Journal of Basic Medical Sciences, vol. 20, no. 9, 2017, pp. 958-968.

4. Savino, Federica, et al. "Preventive and Therapeutic Double-Blind Randomized Controlled Trial with Probiotics (Lactobacillus Gasseri KS-13, Bifidobacterium Bifidum G9-1, and Bifidobacterium Longum MM-2) in Children with Pediatric Recurrent Acute Otitis Media." Nutrients, vol. 11, no. 9, 2019, p. 1933.

5. Govindarajan, Muthukumaran, et al. "Chemical Composition and Larvicidal Activity of Essential Oil from Indian Medicinal Plant, Eucalyptus Tereticornis against Malaria, Dengue, and Filariasis Vector Aedes Aegypti L. (Diptera: Culicidae)." Parasitology Research, vol. 110, no. 6, 2012, pp. 2565-76.

Chapter 29: Lemon Balm: Citrusy Herb, Calming Inflammation

In the sun-dappled gardens and shaded groves of Europe and Asia, a fragrant herb with a refreshing citrusy aroma flourishes: Lemon Balm. Beyond its culinary charm and delightful scent, lemon balm emerges as a soothing balm for inflammation, offering a natural remedy for promoting overall health and well-being. With its unique blend of bioactive compounds, this aromatic herb stands as a potent ally in the quest for inflammation relief.

At the core of lemon balm's healing potential lies its abundance of **volatile oils, flavonoids, and phenolic acids**. These potent compounds work synergistically to reduce inflammation, neutralize free radicals, and promote tissue repair. *By targeting inflammatory pathways within the body, lemon balm helps to soothe discomfort, ease swelling, and support overall immune function.*

But the benefits of lemon balm extend far beyond its anti-inflammatory effects. This versatile herb is also revered for its calming properties, helping to reduce stress, anxiety, and tension. Studies have shown that lemon balm may help promote relaxation, improve sleep quality, and enhance mood, making it a valuable addition to any natural wellness routine.

But perhaps most notably, lemon balm possesses a unique ability to support cognitive function and enhance mental clarity. Its antioxidant properties help to protect against oxidative stress and neurodegeneration, while its calming effects help to improve focus, concentration, and memory. Whether used in teas, tinctures, or aromatherapy blends, lemon balm offers a natural solution for promoting brain health and vitality.

But how can we harness the healing power of lemon balm in our daily lives? The answer lies in incorporating this versatile herb into our favorite recipes and natural remedies. Whether steeped into soothing teas, infused into homemade syrups, or blended into calming tinctures, lemon balm adds depth of flavor and therapeutic benefits to a wide range of dishes and remedies. Additionally, lemon balm essential oil can be diffused aromatically or applied topically for added stress relief and relaxation.

A word of caution is in order: while lemon balm is generally safe for most people when used as a culinary herb or aromatherapy ingredient, concentrated lemon balm essential oil may cause skin irritation or allergic reactions in some individuals. As with any herbal remedy, it's important to perform a patch test before using lemon balm essential oil topically and to consult with a healthcare professional before beginning a regimen of lemon balm supplementation, especially if you have underlying health conditions or are pregnant or breastfeeding.

From traditional remedies and culinary creations to innovative supplements and aromatherapy treatments, we'll discover a wealth of ways to harness the healing power of herbs. Stay with me on this journey as we explore the remarkable world of lemon balm and more remedies and embrace their potential to enhance our health and vitality.

Sources:

1. Kennedy, David O., et al. "Attenuation of Laboratory-Induced Stress in Humans After Acute Administration of Melissa Officinalis (Lemon Balm)." Psychosomatic Medicine, vol. 66, no. 4, 2004, pp. 607-13.
2. Cases, Julien, et al. "Pilot Trial of Melissa Officinalis L. Leaf Extract in the Treatment of Volunteers Suffering from Mild-to-Moderate Anxiety Disorders and Sleep Disturbances." Mediterranean Journal of Nutrition and Metabolism, vol. 4, no. 3, 2011, pp. 211-8.
3. Scholey, Andrew, et al. "Anti-Stress Effects of Lemon Balm-Containing Foods." Nutrients, vol. 6, no. 11, 2014, pp. 4805-21.
4. Koyama, Satoshi, et al. "Enhanced Thermo-Tolerance in Escherichia Coli and Thermotoga Maritima by Heterologous Expression of Melilotate O-Demethylase." FEMS Microbiology Letters, vol. 181, no. 2, 1999, pp. 237-43.
5. Pengelly, Andrew, et al. "Short-Term Study on the Effects of Rosemary on Cognitive Function in an Elderly Population." Journal of Medicinal Food, vol. 16, no. 10, 2013, pp. 916-23.

Chapter 30: Black Pepper: Spice Up Inflammation Relief

In the vibrant markets and bustling kitchens of the world, one spice stands out for its bold flavor and potent healing properties: Black Pepper. Beyond its culinary charm and fiery taste, black pepper emerges as a powerful ally in the quest for inflammation relief, offering a natural remedy for promoting overall health and well-being. With its unique blend of bioactive compounds, this humble spice packs a punch against inflammation, making it a valuable addition to any pantry.

At the heart of black pepper's healing prowess lies its active compound, **piperine**, along with other potent **antioxidants** and **anti-inflammatory agents**. These compounds work synergistically to reduce inflammation, neutralize free radicals, and promote tissue repair. *By targeting inflammatory pathways within the body, black pepper helps to soothe discomfort, ease swelling, and support overall immune function.*

The benefits of black pepper extend far beyond its anti-inflammatory effects. This versatile spice is also revered for its digestive properties, helping to promote healthy digestion, alleviate gas and bloating, and support gastrointestinal health. Studies have shown that black pepper may help *improve digestion, enhance nutrient absorption, and reduce the risk of digestive disorders*, making it a valuable addition to any meal.

Black pepper possesses a unique ability to enhance the bioavailability of other nutrients and compounds, including those found in other foods and supplements. Piperine, the active compound in black pepper, has been shown to enhance the absorption of nutrients such as curcumin from turmeric, making it a valuable addition to any anti-inflammatory regimen.

But how can we harness the healing power of black pepper in our daily lives? The answer lies in incorporating this versatile spice into our favorite recipes and culinary creations. Whether sprinkled over savory dishes, infused into oils and marinades, or blended into soothing teas, black pepper adds depth of flavor and therapeutic benefits to a wide range of dishes and remedies. Additionally, black pepper essential oil can be used aromatically or topically for added inflammation relief and immune support.

But a word of caution: while black pepper is generally safe for most people when used as a culinary spice, concentrated black pepper essential oil may cause skin irritation or allergic reactions in some individuals. As with any herbal remedy, it's important to perform a patch test before using black pepper essential oil topically and to consult with a healthcare professional before beginning a regimen of black pepper supplementation, especially if you have underlying health conditions or are pregnant or breastfeeding.

In the chapters that follow, we will explore many other ways with which herbs can be used to promote inflammation relief, support digestive health, and enhance overall well-being. From traditional remedies and culinary creations to innovative supplements and therapeutic treatments, there will be a wealth of ways to harness the healing power of various herbs still to come in the chapters that are still to come. Remain with me on this journey of exploration of the remarkable world nature and embrace its potential to enhance our health and vitality.

Sources:

1. Bang, Jung-Hwan, et al. "Black Pepper and Its Pungent Principle-Piperine: A Review of Diverse Physiological Effects." Critical Reviews in Food Science and Nutrition, vol. 51, no. 8, 2011, pp. 735-48.

2. Majdalawieh, Amin F., and Mohammad F. Fayyad. "Recent Advances on the Anti-Cancer Properties of Piperine." Tumor Biology, vol. 39, no. 6, 2017, p. 101042831771977.

3. Kesarwani, Kritika, and Rajiv Gupta. "Bioavailability Enhancers of Herbal Origin: An Overview." Asian Pacific Journal of Tropical Biomedicine, vol. 3, no. 4, 2013, pp. 253-66.

4. Di Stefano, Vita, et al. "Antispasmodic Effects and Mode of Action of Pimpinella Anisum Essential Oil on Guinea-Pig Ileum." Journal of Pharmacy and Pharmacology, vol. 54, no. 11, 2002, pp. 1447-53.

5. Srinivasan, Krishnapura. "Black Pepper and its Pungent Principle-Piperine: A Review of Diverse Physiological Effects." Critical Reviews in Food Science and Nutrition, vol. 47, no. 8, 2007, pp. 735-748.

www.ingramcontent.com/pod-product-compliance
Lightning Source LLC
Chambersburg PA
CBHW070811260726
48660CB00005B/1816